May 2
cmc

# HARRIET ROTH'S
# FAT COUNTER

REVISED EDITION

# HARRIET ROTH'S
# FAT COUNTER

## REVISED EDITION

by

## Harriet Roth

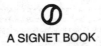

A SIGNET BOOK

SIGNET
Published by New American Library, a division of
Penguin Group (USA) Inc., 375 Hudson Street, New York, New York 10014, USA
Penguin Group (Canada), 90 Eglinton Avenue East, Suite 700, Toronto,
Ontario M4P 2Y3, Canada (a division of Pearson Penguin Canada Inc.)
Penguin Books Ltd., 80 Strand, London WC2R 0RL, England
Penguin Ireland, 25 St. Stephen's Green, Dublin 2, Ireland (a division of Penguin Books Ltd.)
Penguin Group (Australia), 250 Camberwell Road, Camberwell, Victoria 3124,
Australia (a division of Pearson Australia Group Pty. Ltd.)
Penguin Books India Pvt. Ltd., 11 Community Centre, Panchsheel Park, New Delhi - 110 017, India
Penguin Group (NZ), cnr Airborne and Rosedale Roads, Albany,
Auckland 1310, New Zealand (a division of Pearson New Zealand Ltd.)
Penguin Books (South Africa) (Pty.) Ltd., 24 Sturdee Avenue,
Rosebank, Johannesburg 2196, South Africa

Penguin Books Ltd., Registered Offices: 80 Strand, London WC2R 0RL, England

First published by Signet, an imprint of New American Library, a division of Penguin Group (USA) Inc.

First Printing, January 1992
First Printing (Revised Edition), April 1993
First Printing (Second Revised Edition), January 1999
First Printing (Third Revised Edition), January 2007
20 19 18 17 16 15 14 13 12 11

# CONTENTS

# NOTE TO THE READER

This book is not intended as a substitute for medical advice or treatment of specific medical problems.

# ACKNOWLEDGMENTS

Sharon Levine Waldman

Nutritional analysis by WellTech Solutions.

Nutritional information adapted from the following sources:

ESHA Research. The Food Processor SQL. Software. Salem, OR: ESHA Research, 2004–2005.

Hurley, Jayne, and Bonnie Liebman. "Restaurant Roulette." *CSPI Nutrition Action Health Letter* (January-February 2005): 11–15.

Linda McDonald Associates, Inc. "Brand-Name Shopping List." *Supermarket Savvy* (2005).

Peapod (Internet grocer). http://www.peapod.com.

Pennington, Jean A.T., and Judith Spungen Douglass. *Bowes and Church's Food Values of Portions Commonly Used.* 18th ed. Philadelphia: Lippincott Williams & Wilkins, 2004.

U.S. Department of Agriculture, Agricultural Research Service. USDA Nutrient Database for Standard Reference, Release 18. 2005. Nutrient Data Laboratory. http://www.ars.usda.gov/nutrientdata.

Peters, Anne, M.D. *Conquering Diabetes.* New York: Hudson Street Press, Penguin Group USA, 2005.

Special thanks to the many food manufacturers, fast food companies, and Gelson's markets who were so generous with their time and information.

# ARE YOU SABOTAGING YOUR HEALTH?

Answer True or False:
1. You think of "bread and butter" as one word.
2. You think of yourself as a "meat and potatoes" person.
3. Among your favorite comfort foods are commercially prepared baked goods, doughnuts, snack foods, fried foods, stick margarine, and french fries.
4. You avoid whole grains, salads, fresh vegetables, and fruits.
5. You are someone who eats everything you feel like eating, anytime, anyplace.
6. You never miss a chance to have a rich dessert, and feel that no meal is complete without one.
7. You seldom read labels on the foods you buy.
8. You eat at fast-food restaurants at least once a week.
9. Whenever you get the urge to exercise, you relax and wait until the feeling passes.
10. You count on the fact that, if you ever develop diabetes or a coronary problem, there will be a drug or some "medical miracle" to save you.
11. You think the fuss about trans fat is transitory.

## What's Your Score?

If you answered True to:

| | |
|---|---|
| 2 or fewer: | No gold star, but you're on your way! |
| 3 to 4: | Not bad, but there's room for improvement. |
| 5 or more: | Stop! Work on it! And don't be discouraged if you aren't perfect. |

---

The average life expectancy for women is 80 years; for men, it's 74.8—unless you live in Okinawa, where it's 81.2 years, with the highest percentage of people living more than 100 years.

So, if you knew you were going to live so long, would you have taken better care of yourself?

---

# A RECIPE FOR YOUR GOOD HEALTH

### Creating a Healthy Environment

Losing weight is easy—you've done it a hundred times.

Almost two-thirds of Americans are overweight or obese. Rates of obesity among adults and children have doubled in the last 25 years and tripled among teenagers. Two-thirds of the world population is underfed. In the United States, however, most people are overfed and underexercised.

Unfortunately, we live in the computer age, in which many children come home from sitting in school to sit in front of television sets or computers. This behavior establishes a pattern of not exercising.

> **Good nutrition depends on your total diet, not a single food.**

Americans are living longer than ever before. Since we are living longer, it behooves us to address our health.

Each year, more than 50 million Americans are obsessed with going on a diet. Unfortunately, the majority regain the lost pounds, and then some.

The Centers for Disease Control calls obesity "a very important health problem." Our increasingly **sedentary lifestyle** as well as **supersized portions** may be the primary obesity culprits.

Two of the most significant changes you can make in your lifestyle are to **focus on the amount and kind of fat that you eat while limiting your portions**. If you limit the "bad" fats—*trans fats and saturated fats*—and emphasize the "good" fats—olive oil, canola oil, safflower, sunflower, peanut, walnut (vegetable oils that have *not been hydrogenated*)—you will discover a healthier *you* while losing pounds and maintaining your weight loss.

### In Losing Weight, a Little Can Mean a Lot

1. Reduce your portions a bit.
2. Don't have second helpings.
3. Switch to nonfat or 1% fat dairy products.
4. Use "good" fats and limit "bad" fats.
5. Enjoy fresh fruit for dessert instead of the traditional cakes or pies.
6. Eliminate empty calories such as sodas, excessive alcoholic beverages, white bread, and white rice.
7. Do at least 30 minutes of exercise daily.

## Body Mass Index

Experts like to use a measurement called BMI, which stands for body mass index, a measure that relates weight to height, to determine optimal weight for good health. Excess fat in the diet may contribute to heart disease; to cancer of the breast, pancreas, prostate, and colon; and to diabetes.* **A BMI of 20 to 21 is ideal. A BMI higher than 25 indicates an overweight problem. A BMI of 29 or higher indicates obesity.** Based on BMI, at least one-half of all Americans are currently overweight.

## What's Your BMI?

1. Locate your height in the left column.
2. Follow the row across until you find the weight closest to your weight.
3. The number at the top of that column is your BMI. If your weight is less than the first number in the row for your height, your BMI is under 20. If your weight is more than the last number in the row for your height, your BMI is over 30.

| BMI → | Normal | | | | | Overweight | | | | Obese | |
|---|---|---|---|---|---|---|---|---|---|---|---|
| | 20 | 21 | 22 | 23 | 24 | 25 | 26 | 27 | 28 | 29 | 30 |
| **Height** ⇩ | ⇐ **Weight** (pounds) ⇒ | | | | | | | | | | |
| 4'10" | 95 | 100 | 105 | 110 | 114 | 119 | 124 | 129 | 133 | 138 | 143 |
| 4'11" | 99 | 104 | 109 | 114 | 119 | 124 | 129 | 134 | 139 | 144 | 149 |
| 5' | 102 | 107 | 112 | 117 | 122 | 127 | 132 | 138 | 143 | 148 | 153 |
| 5'1" | 106 | 111 | 117 | 122 | 127 | 132 | 138 | 143 | 148 | 154 | 159 |
| 5'2" | 109 | 114 | 120 | 125 | 130 | 136 | 141 | 147 | 152 | 158 | 163 |
| 5'3" | 113 | 119 | 124 | 130 | 135 | 141 | 147 | 152 | 158 | 164 | 168 |
| 5'4" | 117 | 123 | 129 | 135 | 141 | 146 | 152 | 158 | 164 | 170 | 170 |
| 5'5" | 120 | 126 | 132 | 138 | 144 | 150 | 156 | 162 | 168 | 174 | 180 |
| 5'6" | 124 | 131 | 137 | 143 | 149 | 156 | 162 | 168 | 174 | 180 | 187 |
| 5'7" | 127 | 134 | 140 | 147 | 153 | 159 | 166 | 172 | 178 | 185 | 191 |
| 5'8" | 132 | 139 | 145 | 152 | 158 | 165 | 172 | 178 | 185 | 191 | 198 |
| 5'9" | 135 | 142 | 149 | 155 | 162 | 169 | 176 | 182 | 189 | 196 | 203 |
| 5'10" | 140 | 147 | 154 | 161 | 168 | 175 | 182 | 189 | 196 | 203 | 210 |
| 5'11" | 143 | 150 | 157 | 164 | 171 | 179 | 186 | 193 | 200 | 207 | 214 |
| 6' | 148 | 155 | 162 | 170 | 177 | 185 | 192 | 199 | 207 | 214 | 221 |
| 6'1" | 151 | 158 | 166 | 174 | 181 | 189 | 196 | 204 | 211 | 219 | 226 |
| 6'2" | 156 | 164 | 171 | 179 | 187 | 195 | 203 | 210 | 218 | 226 | 234 |

## High Fat, Low Fat, Some Fat, No Fat

Are you confused and overstimulated from too much information about dietary fat and what part it plays in our diet?

Billy Crystal is quoted as saying that he was 13 years old before he realized that his name wasn't "Taste this." The taste for fat is learned from childhood on; however, it can be modified even during adulthood.

*According to Katherine Flegal, Ph.D., National Center for Health Statistics.

But how low should fat go? Some experts say that fat should not make up more than 30% of your calories as long as saturated fats and trans fats combined don't make up more than 10% of your calories.

We recommend the more prudent 20% or less, with emphasis on olive oil and canola oil, and extreme limitation of foods containing saturated fat and trans fat. By eating more fruits, vegetables, cereals, and whole grain products, limiting animal protein (not more than 4 to 5 ounces daily), and avoiding hydrogenated oils, we can easily limit our fat to this percentage. The gain will be in good health—the loss, in weight.

## What's the Skinny on Fat?

We used to think that simply cutting the total amount of calories we ate each day would lead to weight loss. Now we know that it is not just any calories, but specifically fat calories and portions that we must watch. There are 9 calories in every gram of fat, twice as many as in every gram of protein or carbohydrate. **All calories are not created equal!**

To determine your daily allowable calories from fat:

> Approximate calories you consume daily x 20% (.20) = Daily calories allowable from fat.

If you want to lose weight and then maintain your desired weight:

> *Step 1:* Desired weight × 15 calories = Total daily calories needed for optimal weight.
> *Step 2:* Optimal daily calories × 20% (.20) = Total daily calories allowable from fat.

What does this mean in terms of the amount of fat you can eat each day? You need to convert your allowable fat calories into grams:

> Daily allowable calories from fat ÷ 9 (9 calories in 1 gram of fat) = Total grams of fat allowed daily.

## The Daily Fat Target in Grams (20% of Total Daily Calories)

| Daily Calorie Level | Grams of Fat |
|---|---|
| 1200 | 26 |
| 1500 | 33 |
| 1800 | 40 |
| 2000 | 44 |
| 2200 | 49 |
| 2500 | 56 |
| 3000 | 67 |

If your total daily calorie allowance is 1,500, for example, following the 20% guideline would allow you to consume 33 grams of fat a day. Now, most of us have no idea what 33 grams of fat would be. Thirty-three grams of fat is about the equivalent of 6 teaspoons of oil or 8 pats of butter. The average American consumes 80 to 100 grams of fat per day! To help you plan your daily diet and limit your fat, I have given the total grams of fat, saturated fat, trans fat, and total calories for each food listed in this book.

A good rule of thumb to follow for keeping your fat content within the healthful 20% guideline is about 2 grams of fat per 100 calories. Some foods that you eat may have more than 2 grams of fat per 100 calories, while others contain less—for example, fruits, vegetables, grains, and nonfat dairy products. You can figure out the fat/calorie ratio from the listings in this book. Obviously, an occasional high-fat "treat" is not fatal, but remember that one indulgence could be your entire fat allowance or more for the day. For example, a snack of 1/2 cup of oil-roasted peanuts contains 35 grams of fat, your entire fat allowance for the day on a 1500-calorie diet. Remember that the 20% fat content of each food is only a general guideline; it's the total grams of fat and calories consumed daily that count.

### Trans Fat and Saturated Fat—The Dangerous Culprits

> Remember that eating food high in saturated fat and trans fat raises total blood cholesterol levels more than eating dietary cholesterol does.

We know that diets high in saturated fat contribute to heart disease by raising cholesterol levels. All saturated fat raises cholesterol. Saturated fats, which are generally solid at room temperature, are found primarily in foods of animal origin such as whole milk dairy products (butter, cream, milk, sour cream, ice cream, and cheeses), and in meat, lard, chicken, and beef fat. Saturated fats also are found in tropical oils such as coconut oil, palm oil, palm kernel oil, cocoa butter, and *any vegetable oil that has been hydrogenated*, such as solid vegetable shortening and stick margarine. Remember, the softer the margarine, the less saturated fat it contains. However, **when any oil is hydrogenated, it becomes more solid and saturated, and it also forms trans fat**. It is thus more likely to raise your cholesterol level. Tropical oils (e.g., palm or coconut oil) and hydrogenated fats are used commercially because they are inexpensive and the process increases the shelf life and flavor stability of the foods. But this resulting trans fat, like saturated fat, also **raises the low-density lipoprotein (LDL, bad cholesterol) in the blood**. Moreover, **unlike saturated fat, trans fat *lowers* high-density lipoprotein (HDL, good cholesterol) in the blood**.

Nothing in our food supply is more dangerous than trans-fatty acids (trans fat). "By our most conservative estimate, replacement of partially hydrogenated fat in the U.S. diet with **natural unhydrogenated vegetable oils** would prevent approximately 30,000 premature coronary deaths per year, and epidemiologic evidence suggests this number is closer to 100,000 premature deaths annually," according to the Harvard School of Public Health.

Dr. Walter Willett, chairman of the Department of Nutrition at the Harvard School of Public Health, calls the partial hydrogenation of oils "the biggest food processing disaster in United States history."

---

Where Will I Find Trans Fat?
  Vegetable shortenings, stick margarines, crackers, cakes, cookies, donuts, french fries, snack foods, and other foods made with or fried in partially hydrogenated oils.

---

Trying to count saturated fat, trans fat, and total fat can get to be a burden that can be discouraging. Counting total fat is simple! If you limit your total fat to 20% of your calories, you will automatically be limiting your saturated fat intake. However, remember, **saturated fat and trans fat together should make up no more than 10% of your total fat calories**. For your information, I have provided a separate listing of saturated fat and newly labeled trans fat for the foods in this book for which information is available at this time.

We consume relatively small amounts of trans fat compared to saturated fat, but **trans fat's impact is large**. Small amounts of trans fats occur naturally in foods of animal origin, but most of the trans fat we eat comes from **hydrogenated vegetable oils used in processed foods**, such as vegetable shortening, stick margarine, store-bought cakes, cookies, crackers, fried foods from fast-food chains and restaurants, and supermarket frozen foods. Nondairy creamers, flavored coffees, and whipped toppings also contain trans fat.

Food manufacturers are presently changing nutrition facts labels to list the amounts of trans fat in their products. This labeling change applies to all packaged foods that enter interstate commerce in the United States as of January 1, 2006. However, a food may contain up to 0.5 milligrams of trans fat per serving and the manufacturer may still list it on the label as "0 mg. trans fat." Be wary: If major entries in the ingredient list are "partially hydrogenated" or "hydrogenated" oils, a serving could contain up to 0.4 milligrams of trans fat—adding up quickly if you have several servings!

Dietary supplement manufacturers must also list trans fat on the nutrition facts panel when their product contains trans fat. Examples of supplements containing trans fat are some **energy and nutrition bars**.

## The American Heart Association's
## Updated Dietary Recommendations Issued in 2006

The AHA now says that trans fats should make up just 1 percent or less of your total daily calories. For example, on 2000 calories daily, that's about two grams of transfat per day (approximately half of a small bag of the average fast-food fries).

To summarize, the following are recommendations for a permanent healthy lifestyle.

1. Consider increasing daily physical activity.
2. Stop smoking.
3. Trim the saturated fat to 7 percent of total calories and limit trans fats to 1 percent of total calories.
4. Use low-fat dairy products and lean cuts of meat, and eat smaller portions.
5. Include more vegetables and fruits daily.
6. Eat two fish meals per week. Best choices are oily fish, high in healthful omega-3 fatty acids, such as herring, sardines, salmon, lake trout, mackerel, and albacore tuna.
7. Avoid foods made with hydrogenated or partially hydrogenated fat.
8. Eat cereal, bread, crackers, and pastas that are whole grain and high fiber—at least 6 servings per day.
9. Soy foods are recommended to replace high-fat animal products; however, soy will not reduce blood cholesterol or other heart-related risk factors.

### Major Food Sources of Trans Fat in the American Diet

(average daily trans fat intake is 5.8 grams, or 2.6% of calories)

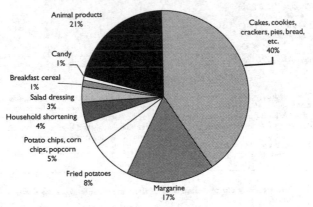

Source: U.S. Food and Drug Administration.

To lower your intake of saturated fat, trans fat, and cholesterol, compare similar foods and choose those with lower **combined** saturated and trans fats and lower cholesterol.

### Total Fat, Saturated Fat, Trans Fat and Cholesterol Content Per Serving

| Product | Common Serving Size | Total Fat Grams | Saturated Fat Grams | % Daily Value for Saturated Fat | Trans Fat Grams | Combined Saturated and Trans Fat | Cholesterol (mg.) |
|---|---|---|---|---|---|---|---|
| French fries (fast food) | Medium (147 grams) | 27 | 7 | 35 | 8 | 15 | 0 |
| Butter | 1 tb. | 11 | 7 | 35 | 0 | 7 | 30 |
| Margarine, stick | 1 tb. | 11 | 2 | 10 | 3 | 5 | 0 |
| Margarine, tub | 1 tb. | 7 | 1 | 5 | 0.5 | 1.5 | 0 |
| Mayonnaise (soybean oil) | 1 tb. | 11 | 1.5 | 8 | 0 | 1.5 | 5 |
| Shortening | 1 tb. | 13 | 3.5 | 18 | 4 | 7.5 | 0 |
| Potato chips | Small bag (42.5 g.) | 11 | 2 | 10 | 3 | 5 | 0 |
| Milk, whole | 1 cup | 7 | 4.5 | 23 | 0 | 4.5 | 35 |
| Milk, skim | 1 cup | 0 | 0 | 0 | 0 | 0 | 5 |
| Doughnut | 1 | 18 | 4.5 | 23 | 5 | 9.5 | 25 |
| Cookies (cream filled) | 3 (30 g.) | 6 | 1 | 5 | 2 | 3 | 0 |
| Candy bar | 1 (40 g.) | 10 | 4 | 20 | 3 | 7 | < 5 |
| Cake, pound | 1 slice (80 g.) | 16 | 3.5 | 18 | 4.5 | 8 | 0 |

Nutrient values based on the U.S. Food and Drug Administration's nutrition labeling regulations.

### How to Avoid Trans Fat

One hundred years ago, it was much simpler to avoid trans fat because of the foods that were—and were not—available. Today, because of ever-increasing consumption of take-out foods, packaged and convenience foods, restaurant and fast foods, cookies, doughnuts, french fries, cakes, crackers, chips, certain cereals, and even some "nutrition bars" or supplements, we are subject to higher trans fat levels. **Your goal is to have as little trans fat in your diet as possible**.

So how do we limit our intake of trans fat?

---

**Americans get more than 35% of their calories dining away from home.**

---

- Read your label for a listing of trans fat and look for partially hydrogenated or hydrogenated oil as one of the ingredients. If one of them is present, choose another product.
- Use a more healthful spread. The softer a margarine, the better—it means it is lower in trans fat. Look for one that is **labeled "trans fat free."**
- Choose olive oil or canola oil instead of margarine or butter, and certainly choose olive or canola oil for any frying or sautéing.
- We live in a busy time, but try to opt for more healthful home cooking.
- "Do not switch from trans fat to saturated fat. Your aim should be to minimize the intake of both," advises Alice H. Lichtenstein, Stanley N. Gershoff Professor of Nutrition Science and Policy at Tufts University's Friedman School of Nutrition Science and Policy.
- If you understand the danger of trans fat, if you read labels carefully and avoid restaurant and bakery-baked goods, nondairy creamers, and fried foods—IF YOU UNDERSTAND THAT YOU HAVE OPTIONS—you will enjoy a healthier and longer life.

### The New Nutrition Facts Label

Accurate food labels are critical for millions of consumers who are overweight, have diabetes, high blood pressure, or food allergies, or are on restricted diets that require careful monitoring of fats, carbohydrates, sugar, and calories that they consume.

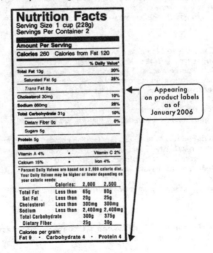

Ingredients: Enriched (*wheat*) flour, malted barley, sugar, whey (*milk*), eggs, vanilla, lecithin (*soy*). *Contains wheat, milk, and soy.*

# A More Complete Label—At Last!

### Trans Fat

**In 1994, the Center for Science in the Public Interest (CSPI), a consumer advocacy organization,** filed a petition with the U.S. Food and Drug Administration (FDA) requesting that the agency take steps to require that trans fat be listed on nutrition labels and claims. In 1999, the FDA amended its regulations to require that trans fat be listed on nutrition labels. On January 1, 2006, new federal food labeling requirements went into effect to include trans fats—the new kid on the block. The FDA is *not banning food manufacturers from using trans fat* in packaged foods. The FDA *is* requiring food manufacturers, processors, and distributors **to label the amount of trans fat in a serving of food** on the nutrition facts panel. As a result, consumers will have information they need to reduce their intake of trans fat.

### Allergens

Also effective January 1, 2006, the FDA requires food labels to clearly state whether a food product contains any protein derived from the eight major allergenic foods: milk, eggs, fish, crustacean shellfish, tree nuts, peanuts, wheat, and soybeans. In the ingredient list, manufacturers must add the common name of the product so the consumer clearly knows whether it contains possible allergens. Manufacturers must also state which allergens it contains in a separate line. In the label displayed, the words in italics were added to comply with the new law.

### New Label Language

- **Calorie free:** No more than 5 calories per serving.
- **Sugar free:** Less than ½ gram of sugar per serving.
- **Salt free:** Fewer than 5 milligrams of sodium per serving.
- **Low sodium:** No more than 140 milligrams of sodium per serving.
- **Fat free:** Less than ½ gram of fat per serving, provided the food has no added fat or oil ingredients.
- **Low fat:** No more than 3 grams of fat per serving.
- **Light:** Either ⅓ fewer calories than, or half the fat in, the regular version of a similar food.
- **Reduced fat:** At least 25% less fat than comparison food.
- **Low in saturated fat:** No more than 1 gram of saturated fat per serving and no more than 15% of its calories from saturated fat.
- **Reduced saturated fat:** No more than 50% of the saturated fat of comparison food.
- **Trans Fats:** 0.5 grams or less may be indicated as "0" trans fat.

*A WORD OF CAUTION:* **When fat content in processed foods is reduced, sodium or sugar content is generally increased. Check your food labels.**

## Nutrition Facts

Labels are now required to carry a chart of standard nutritional information that:

1. Requires more realistic and consistent serving information.
2. Lists total calories plus calories from fat based on the theory that people should get no more than 30% of calories from fat.
3. Gives the percent daily value, showing how the food fits into overall nutritional requirements.
4. Lists nutrients most important to good health based on a balanced diet of 2,000 or 2,500 calorie daily intake.
5. Lists number of calories per gram of fat (9), carbohydrates (4), and protein (4).

**Fast-food restaurants are not required to have nutrition labels; however, they will provide nutrition information if requested.**

### What Is Cholesterol and Where Do We Get It?

Dietary cholesterol is a fatty, waxlike substance that **can be found only in foods of animal origin.** A food can be high in fat—for instance, nuts, avocados, or chocolate—but contain no cholesterol. That is because these foods originate from plant, not animal, sources. Some foods are high in cholesterol—such as shellfish—but low in saturated fat. Saturated fat raises cholesterol more than the cholesterol found in food does.

> **Cholesterol levels don't just come from food; they come from our genes.**

To help prevent heart disease, the American Heart Association suggests an allowance of no more than 100 milligrams of cholesterol for every 1,000 calories that you consume per day, up to a maximum of 300 milligrams. You can do this by eating more whole grains, fruits, and vegetables, limiting your portion of any animal protein to 4 to 5 ounces per day, and having 2 to 3 days per week that are completely vegetarian.

> **Lean meat has as much cholesterol as fatty meat.**

About 75% of our cholesterol is manufactured by the liver, and the rest is obtained from the foods that we eat. We cannot control our genetic tendencies to manufacture cholesterol, but we can control our food habits. Cholesterol comes in two forms in the body: HDL, or good cholesterol, and LDL, or bad cholesterol. LDL has been linked to the buildup of plaque in the walls of the coronary arteries. This plaque can result in a heart attack or stroke. Prime sources of dietary cholesterol are found in foods from animal sources, and we must also limit consumption of foods containing saturated fats, such as meat, poultry (especially the skin), cheeses, whole milk, butter, and ice cream, since they raise cholesterol levels. The other culprit is **trans fat,** found in coconut and palm oils, and all hydrogenated fats. **Trans fats raise LDL levels and lower HDL levels.**

Cholesterol Basics

The National Institutes of Health categorizes cholesterol levels in the following way:

**Total Cholesterol Level**

| | | |
|---|---|---|
| | Less than 200 mg/dL | Desirable |
| | 200–239 mg/dL | Borderline high |
| | 240 mg/dL and above | High |

**LDL Cholesterol Level**

| | | |
|---|---|---|
| | Less than 100 mg/dL | Optimal |
| | 100–129 mg/dL | Near optimal |
| | 130–159 mg/dL | Borderline high |
| | 160 and above | High |

**HDL Cholesterol Level**

| | | |
|---|---|---|
| | Less than 50 mg/dL | Low |
| | 60 mg/dL and above | Desirable |

Remember, you want your HDL level to be high, and your LDL level to be low. An elevated LDL cholesterol increases the risk of developing coronary heart disease.

Additionally, people who have triglyceride levels that are borderline high (150–199 milligrams per deciliter) or high (200 milligrams per deciliter or more) may need medical treatment.

These test results also carry a determination of the **heart-risk ratio: the ratio of HDL to total cholesterol.** This ratio is obtained by dividing the total cholesterol count by the HDL count. **The ideal number for this ratio is 4.5 or lower.** For example, if your total cholesterol is 180, and your HDL is 50, your heart-risk ratio would be 3.6.

The next time you visit your physician and have a blood panel, request that you receive a hard copy of your results so that you can "know your numbers."

---

**Know Your Numbers**

Knowing your total cholesterol is not enough.
Blood pressure: 120/80 mmHg or less
Blood glucose (fasting): less than 110 mg/dL
Total cholesterol: 200 mg/dL or less
CRP (C-reactive protein)*: 0.000–0.400
LDL: 100 mg/dL (or less with risk factors)
HDL: 50 mg/dL or more
AIC: less than 6% (6% or more indicates prediabetes)
BMI: 18–24.9
Waist circumference: less than 35" women; less than 40" men

---

\* CRP (high-sensitive C-reactive protein) is a powerful predictor of cardiovascular disease and type 2 diabetes.

## Omega-3 Fatty Acid Levels in Fish

The American Heart Association contends that for older men and women the benefits of eating fish far outweigh the risk of contaminants. Fish is a good source of protein and is low in saturated fat. Two to three servings of fish per week will provide the necessary heart protection.

To reduce contaminants in fish, remove skin and fat before eating. Larger fish—swordfish, king mackerel, shark, tilefish, golden bass, tuna, and golden snapper—contain higher levels of mercury. Up to 7 ounces a week of these types of fish is acceptable.

An important nutrient found in fish is omega-3 fatty acids—1 gram per day has been shown to have heart-protective benefits. The highest concentration of omega-3 fatty acids is found in the oiliest fish—mackerel, arctic char, sardines, herring, bluefish, and salmon. The amount of fish needed to equal the recommended daily average of 1 gram of omega-3 fatty acids varies with the age of the fish, its diet, and other factors. A form of omega-3 fatty acids (alpha-linolenic acid) is found in canola oil, soy oil, flax seed, and walnuts. Although this form is less effective, it may be valuable to people who do not eat fish.

| Type of Fish | Ounces of Fish Needed to Obtain 1 Gram of Omega-3 Fatty Acids |
|---|---|
| Herring | 1.5–2 |
| Sardines | 2–3 |
| Atlantic salmon, farmed | 2–3.5 |
| Atlantic salmon, wild | 2–8.5 |
| Mackerel | 2–8.5 |
| Tuna (preferably white) | 2.5–15 |
| Coho salmon | 3 |
| Trout | 3–3.5 |
| Swordfish | 4 |
| Sole | 7 |
| Shrimp | 11 |
| Cod | 12.5–23 |

Canned fish (tuna, salmon, and sardines) is also a good source of omega-3 fatty acids. However, with sodium and mercury content as possible concerns, **limit your servings to two to three times per week**.

## It's the Quality of Your Carbohydrates That Counts

Carbohydrates come in two basic forms:

1. **Complex carbohydrates**, or starches, are whole grain breads, cereals, pasta, brown rice, and potatoes. Fruits, vegetables, milk, and yogurt are mostly carbohydrates. Raw fruits and vegetables are also high in fiber, so sugar is more slowly absorbed. Dairy products also contain protein and fat; thus, they are absorbed more slowly.
2. **Simple carbohydrates** are found in sugar and candy. They all ultimately break down into glucose or simple sugar and are immediately absorbed by your bloodstream.

## Can You Find the Carbohydrates?

Check the 9 foods listed below that contain carbohydrates.

_____olive oil
_____skim milk
_____grapes
_____oat bran cereal
_____sausage pizza
_____poached eggs
_____whole wheat bagel
_____carrots
_____bacon
_____black-eyed peas
_____sour cream
_____ground beef
_____corn
_____instant rice

The 9 foods that contain carbohydrates are skim milk, grapes, oat bran cereal, sausage pizza, whole wheat bagel, carrots, black-eyed peas, corn, and instant rice.

---

**One tablespoon of sugar has the same number of calories as a 3-ounce baked potato.**

---

## Sugar

The USDA estimates that the average American eats about 100 pounds of added sugar a year (up 30% since 1980). This enormous intake of sugar in soft drinks and processed foods is partly to blame for the expanding American waistline.

Whole or unprocessed foods, such as fruits, vegetables, and milk, contain natural sugars. However, processed or prepared foods frequently contain added sugars that contribute added calories and few vitamins or minerals.

Recently, the American Diabetes Association (ADA) relaxed its previous restrictions on sugar intake for diabetics. This change was based on the fact that when eaten in the same amount, sweets and complex carbohydrates often affect blood glucose levels similarly. However, a small amount of sugar equals a large amount of carbohydrates. For example, 1 tablespoon of sugar has the same number of calories as a 3-ounce baked potato. In addition, sugar usually keeps bad company, that is, saturated and trans fats found in cakes, cookies, pies, and pastries. By itself, it has empty calories devoid of vitamins, minerals, or fiber. It is preferable for people with diabetes to avoid sugar-containing foods. The FDA has approved artificial sweeteners such as sucralose, aspartame, and saccharine.

**Sugar appears on labels under many different names: syrup, sucrose, dextrose, maltose, lactose, invert sugar, honey, high fructose corn syrup, fructose, fruit juice concentrate, corn syrup, corn sweetener, sugar alcohol, and others.**

Your body converts starch in complex carbohydrates into sugar, which is then absorbed by your bloodstream. Your liver is a very busy organ; it manufactures 75% of your cholesterol, and it also stores simple sugars. It releases them into your bloodstream when needed. Protein replaces carbohydrates as the principal source of sugar also when needed.

> What magical machines our bodies are! Let's not abuse them but appreciate them by choosing a healthy eating plan we can live with. In return, we will be rewarded with increased longevity and the good health to enjoy it.

### Diabetes

Worldwide, between 100 million and 120 million people are troubled by a chronic condition known as diabetes. In the United States, the number currently stands at about 16 million people; nearly half of them do not know yet that they have the disease. More than 3 million are aged 65 or older.

> People of African American, Hispanic or Latino, Native American, Asian American, or Pacific Island ethnicity are more likely to get diabetes.

The ADA divides diabetes into two categories:

**Type 1 diabetes** usually starts before age 30 and tends to come on suddenly.

**Type 2 diabetes,** far more common, usually starts after the age of 30. The majority of those with type 2 diabetes are obese, its onset is more gradual, and blood glucose levels are more stable. Patients may notice few or no symptoms for years. Today, insulin treatment is widely used for both types of diabetes, often in conjunction with oral medications.

> **People of Latino or African American origin are at very high risk for developing diabetes.**

Today's children are overfed and underexercised, resulting in childhood obesity and type 2 diabetes that has reached epidemic proportions. Unless we turn this trend around now, our children may have a shorter rather than longer life expectancy than we now pursue as adults.

Worldwide studies have proven that **diet and exercise can prevent the development of type 2 diabetes** by about half. People who lowered their fat to between 20% and 25% of their caloric intake and walked 30 to 45 minutes 5 times a week were most successful in weight reduction and possibly avoiding type 2 diabetes.

> **One serving of avocado contains 12 grams of fiber.**

## Diet and Diabetes

- Eating the right diet not only may help keep glucose levels in check, but also may help to control factors that affect the development of diabetic complications such as obesity, elevated cholesterol, triglycerides, and high blood pressure.
- According to most experts, people with diabetes should eat a high-carbohydrate, low-fat diet: 60% of calories from carbohydrates and less than 30% (preferably 20%) from fat.
- For diabetics as well as for everyone else, it is important to control total calories, saturated fat, trans fat, and cholesterol, as well as limit protein intake to no more than 25% of total calories.
- Weight loss is important if you are overweight; check your body mass index (BMI) and waist circumference. **The best way to lose weight is by decreasing your calories and portions and increasing your exercise.**
- Dietary fiber slows the absorption of sugars into the bloodstream from the intestine, so a whole orange (almost 4 grams of fiber) is better for you than a glass of orange juice (less than ½ gram of fiber).
- Soluble fiber found in oats, oat bran, legumes, barley, citrus fruits, and apples can help lower blood glucose as well as cholesterol. Insoluble fiber found in whole grains, buckwheat, vegetables, and fruits helps to prevent constipation. Both types of fiber are needed for a healthy diet (about 20 to 25 grams of fiber per day).
- No single diet approach meets everyone's needs.

## Facts About Diabetes

According to the AHA:
- Aim for a healthful blood glucose level of less than 100 milligrams measured after an overnight fast.
- Weighing too much contributes to abnormal blood sugar.
- Diabetes is the number one cause of new blindness.
- Diabetes is the major cause of kidney failure, nerve damage, and amputations.
- Insulin injections are not a cure—but a life-preserving necessity for many people.
- Coronary heart disease is the leading cause of death in people with diabetes.
- Diabetes is the sixth leading cause of death.
- Diabetes is a leading cause of peripheral neuropathy.
- Childhood obesity and type 2 diabetes have reached epidemic proportions.

> Hypoglycemia indicates low blood glucose. It results from a blood sugar level below 70 mg. Missing a meal or snacks can cause hypoglycemia. To boost hypoglycemic blood levels, quickly take ½ to ¾ cup of orange juice or 5 to 7 hard candies (such as LifeSavers) or glucose pills. People with diabetes should always have one of these on hand. Avoid using chocolate or nuts, which contain carbohydrates but take longer to digest because they also contain fat.

## Myths and Misconceptions About Diabetes

**True or False?**

1. Eating too much sugar causes diabetes.
2. People with diabetes should avoid exercise and take it easy. Being active can make your diabetes worse.
3. People with diabetes can tell if their blood glucose levels are too high or too low by the way they feel. But the most accurate way to know is to test it on a home monitor.
4. Diabetes may be caused by a stressful time or event.
5. Chronic complications of diabetes are not inevitable.
6. Only type 1 diabetics use insulin.
7. A diet high in simple sugars is not considered healthful.
8. High-sugar foods often tend to be high-fat foods.
9. Diabetes professionals now consider sugar just another form of carbohydrate that can be enjoyed in moderation when included in your healthful meal plan.
10. People whose diabetes is well controlled and who do not have other health problems or take medicines that restrict their use of alcohol can drink limited amounts of alcohol.
11. Exactly how much a certain food raises blood glucose varies from person to person.
12. Foods that contain carbohydrates such as grains, vegetables, fruit, milk, and sugar have the most immediate impact on blood sugar levels.

Answers: 1. F; 2. F; 3. T; 4. F; 5. T; 6. F; 7. T; 8. T; 9. T; 10. F; 11. T; 12. T.

## Glycemic Index

A recent study found that a diet based on low glycemic index foods reduced body fat and risk factors for diabetes and heart disease. One way to assess carbohydrate quality is the glycemic index. **The glycemic index is the speed with which the sugar in foods is absorbed by the body.** Foods with a high glycemic index enter the bloodstream rapidly, causing a rapid increase in insulin and a sudden drop in blood sugar.

Low glycemic foods promote a slower release of glucose and therefore lessen the rise in insulin and help suppress your appetite and reduce cravings. Go easy on the high glycemic foods (simple sugars, refined flours, and starchy vegetables: corn, peas, and white potatoes) and emphasize low glycemic carbohydrates in your diet. This is only a yardstick for healthy eating.

> **Americans spend about 15 cents out of every food dollar on fruits and vegetables.**

## The Glycemic Index of Selected Carbohydrates

| Food | Glycemic Index |
|------|----------------|
| Instant rice | 91 |
| Baked potato | 85 |
| Corn flakes | 84 |
| Carrots | 71 |
| White bread | 70 |
| Rye bread | 65 |
| Muesli | 56 |
| Banana | 53 |
| Spaghetti | 41 |
| Apple | 36 |
| Lentils | 29 |
| Milk | 27 |
| Peanuts | 14 |
| Broccoli | — |

The database for the glycemic index is www.glycemicindex.com.

### Low glycemic index = less than 50

- Most fruits except tropical and dried fruits
- All vegetables except corn
- Sweet potato
- Beans and peas
- Whole wheat and soba pastas
- Oatmeal
- Sprouted grain and rye breads, whole wheat pita bread, whole wheat tortillas
- Peanuts

> **Americans spend about 19 cents out of every food dollar on candy, gum, soda pop, and bakery items.**

### High glycemic index = more than 70

- White bread
- Baked potato, white rice, and corn
- Instant rice
- **Fruit juices and sweetened jams and jellies**
- Milk and yogurt
- Most cold cereals
- Pretzels
- Snack foods and other foods made with refined flour

> **We need 20 to 25 grams of fiber per day.**

## To Eat Better-Quality Carbohydrates

- Have high-fiber cereal or whole grains for breakfast. Fiber is a carbohydrate that is not converted to sugar in the bloodstream. Adults should try to consume 25 to 30 grams of fiber per day.
- Legumes (beans, peas, and nuts) are loaded with soluble fiber, which slows the rise in blood sugar after a meal.
- Enjoy fruits and vegetables; they're generally low calorie if not always low glycemic index.
- Try mashed yams instead of mashed potatoes.
- Choose snacks wisely; look at their calorie and fat content as well as grams of carbohydrates and sugar (see listings in this book).

## Pass on the Salt and Bring on the Veggies and Fruits

As many as 65 million Americans age 6 and older have high blood pressure. Thirty percent of people with high blood pressure don't know they have it.

According to recent government data, nearly one-third of American adults now have high blood pressure—about 65 million. This is a major risk factor in two of the leading causes of death in this country: heart disease and stroke.

**The percentage of adults with optimal blood pressure drops after age 50.**

The federal government, American Heart Association, and World Health Organizations have all recommended that people cut down on the use of salt and processed foods to prevent or treat high blood pressure. **Another enormous source of foods high in sodium are fast food and take-out restaurants.** Some of their offerings are lower in fat but still very high in sodium.

The link between blood pressure and sodium intake is even stronger than originally noted, especially in middle-aged and older people. Excess salt also increases the risk of osteoporosis and kidney stones by increasing calcium excretion, and there is evidence that it increases risk of asthma, stomach cancer, and heart enlargement.

By the age of 60, more than half of all Americans have hypertension—much of it undiagnosed.

## Control Your Blood Pressure As You Age

> The higher your blood pressure, the higher your risk of heart attack and stroke.

Two out of 10 people in their forties have blood pressure high enough to treat with drugs; 5 out of 10 in their sixties; and 6 out of 10 age 70 or older. Blood-pressure-lowering drugs have side effects and are expensive, so it is preferable to control your blood pressure with lifestyle changes as well.

> **More African Americans than Caucasians have hypertension.**

1. Limit sodium to less than 1,500 milligrams daily. Check labels and avoid foods with more than 480 milligrams of sodium per serving.
2. Lose excess weight (check your BMI; page xi). As little as 5 to 7 pounds can make a difference.
3. Walk, swim, or cycle for 30 to 45 minutes 5 times per week.
4. Limit alcohol to 1 drink per day.
5. Get more potassium and magnesium by eating an assortment of 8 to 10 servings of fruits and veggies daily. (A banana, orange, or potato daily helps increase potassium.)

*Salt substitutes* containing potassium chloride may be harmful to some people. Consult a physician before using a salt substitute.

Changing to a low-salt diet will lower your blood pressure. Even if you do not yet have hypertension, it is certainly in your best interest to prevent it by reducing your sodium intake while your blood pressure is still normal.

The **recommended daily maximum sodium intake is 2,300 milligrams**, or about the equivalent of 1 teaspoon of salt. Individuals with hypertension, African Americans, middle-aged adults, and older adults should aim to consume **no more than 1,500 milligrams of sodium per day**.

About 75% of the salt we eat comes from processed foods and fast foods. Foods high in sodium include canned goods, cold cuts, cheeses, condiments, crackers, snack foods, frozen foods, pickles, salted nuts, and monosodium glutamate (MSG).

### It's the Little Things in Life That Count

The safe and adequate daily range for sodium intake is considered to be 1,100 to 2,300 milligrams for healthy adults. But people watching their intake of salt are often unaware that using condiments, sauces, relishes, and processed foods can add substantial amounts of sodium to their diets (salt is 40% sodium). The following U.S. Department of Agriculture figures illustrate the sodium content of the more popular "extras."

## Sodium Content of Various Seasonings*

| Condiment/Relishes | Amount | Sodium (mg.) |
|---|---|---|
| Garlic powder | 1 tsp. | 1 |
| Garlic salt | 1 tsp. | 1850 |
| Horseradish, prepared | 1 tsp. | 40 |
| Ketchup | 1 tb. | 190 |
| Meat tenderizer | 1 tsp. | 1750 |
| monosodium glutamate (MSG) | 1 tsp. | 492 |
| Mustard, prepared | 1 tsp. | 70 |
| Olives, green | 4 | 323 |
| Onion powder | 1 tsp. | 1 |
| Onion salt | 1 tsp. | 1620 |
| Pickle, dill | 1 (2 oz.) | 928 |
| Pickle, sweet | 1 (½ oz.) | 128 |
| Relish, sweet | 1 tb. | 140 |
| Salt | 1 tsp. | 1938 |
| **Sauces** | | |
| Barbecue | 1 tb. | 130 |
| Chili | 1 tb. | 227 |
| Light soy | 1 tb. | 575 |
| Soy | 1 tb. | 1029 |
| Tabasco | 1 tsp. | 24 |
| Tartar | 1 tb. | 182 |
| Teriyaki | 1 tb. | 690 |
| Worcestershire | 1 tb. | 265 |

*Values for specific foods vary according to brand.

Because of public demand, some of these foods now come in no-salt or reduced-sodium and low-sodium versions. Why is salt so widely used in foods? Because it allows food processors to provide taste in otherwise flavorless packaged foods and to use cheaper ingredients. It also caters to the consumer's palate, which has become accustomed to eating overly salted foods. Some experts feel that salt is the most dangerous food additive.

If you are already eating a heart-healthy, cancer-preventive diet rich in vegetables, fruits, and whole grains and low in fat, chances are it will also be low in sodium. Such a diet has been found to lower blood pressure as effectively as some drugs, according to the DASH program. In controlling hypertension, smaller portion sizes, good nutrition, and regular exercise are still the most important parts of maintaining a healthy lifestyle.

> **"Eat breakfast like a king, lunch like a prince, but eat dinner like a pauper."—Adele Davis**

**Relative Amounts of Dietary Sodium in the American Diet**

**Are you aware of the many different sources of dietary sodium?**

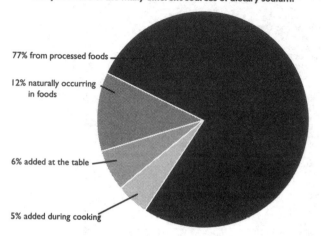

77% from processed foods —

12% naturally occurring in foods

6% added at the table —

5% added during cooking

Graph: FDA. Based on data from the *Journal of the American College of Nutrition*, volume 10, issue 4 (383–393). Copyright © 1991 by American College of Nutrition.

## The DASH Diet

The DASH eating pattern was originally designed to prevent and treat high blood pressure. However, with the passage of time, we have found that the DASH diet is an example of a balanced eating plan consistent with the 2005 dietary guidelines. You don't necessarily have to suffer from high blood pressure to benefit from the DASH diet. It is a well-balanced, easy-to-understand way of eating that can help you:

- Lose weight sensibly
- Lower your cholesterol
- Eat healthier
- **Lower your blood pressure**

Here are the number of servings you should consume daily from each food group. Serving amounts are based on a diet of 2,000 calories per day. Women should consume about 1,500 calories per day.

| Food/Servings | I Serving Equals | Food Examples |
|---|---|---|
| Grains & grain products 7 to 8 a day | I slice bread<br>½ cup dry cereal<br>½ cup cooked brown rice, pasta, or cereal | Whole wheat breads, English muffins, pita bread, cereals, oatmeal, brown rice, corn tortillas, pasta (whole wheat) |
| Fruits 4 to 5 a day | I medium fruit<br>6 oz. fruit juice<br>¼ cup dried, fresh, frozen, or canned fruit | Apricots, blueberries, bananas, strawberries, apples, pears, oranges, grapefruit, melons, peaches, mangos, prunes |
| Vegetables 4 to 5 a day | I cup raw vegetables<br>½ cup any cooked veggies<br>6 oz. vegetable juice | Broccoli, beans, carrots, peas, squash, kale, spinach, sweet potato, tomatoes, all leafy greens |
| Dairy foods (low-fat or nonfat) 2 to 3 a day | 8 oz. milk<br>I cup yogurt<br>I½ oz. cheese | Skim or 1% milk, nonfat or low-fat yogurt, nonfat or part-skim cheese |
| Meats, poultry, & fish No more than 2 a day | 3 oz. cooked meat, poultry, or fish | Lean meats only; trim visible fat; broil, roast, or boil skinless poultry |
| Nuts, seeds, & legumes 4 to 5 a week | ⅓ cup nuts<br>2 tsp. seeds<br>½ cup cooked legumes | Almonds, peanuts, cashews, walnuts, sunflower seeds, kidney beans, lentils, black beans, pinto beans |

*Source:* DASH clinical study, the Mayo Clinic.

---

**Romaine lettuce has 6 times as much vitamin A as iceberg lettuce.**

---

Three to 4 weeks after you stop eating a high-sodium diet, you will find that foods you used to love taste unpleasantly salty and you'll discover that many foods have flavors that taste better than ever. Their naturally delicious qualities are no longer masked with the overpowering characteristics of overly salted foods.

### Losing Weight Is Not a Losing Proposition

Each year more than 50 million Americans are obsessed with going on a diet. Unfortunately, the majority regain the lost pounds, and then some. **The most significant change that you can make in your lifestyle is to reduce the food portions that you eat and count the grams of trans fat and saturated fat.** If you simply reduce your "bad" fat intake and eat moderate portions, weight loss will follow. (The "good" fats are olive, canola, safflower, sunflower, peanut, walnut—vegetable oils that have *not been hydrogenated*.) You will discover that losing weight **and maintaining weight loss** is not just a fad, but an important lifestyle improvement. Not only will you look better; you'll feel better, be more productive, and ultimately be happier.

> **"Thou shouldst eat to live, not live to eat."—Socrates**

## Twelve Choices for Cutting Fat and Calories

1. Count your grams of fat, eat less **(watch your portions)**, and reduce your total calories by about 300 calories per day.
2. Keep a daily food diary. Record everything that passes your lips and check to find out what, when, and why you eat.
3. Keep problem foods out of the house. Limit your low-fat sweets and empty calories such as white bread, pastries, and sodas.
4. Check food labels for total fat, saturated fat, trans fat, carbohydrates, sugar, fiber, and calories.
5. Don't skip meals. Have three meals a day and two snacks. DO NOT GO HUNGRY! Choose low-fat snacks, such as air-popped popcorn, vegetables, fruits, nonfat yogurt, or nonfat crackers and low-fat cheese.

> **Broccoli florets are more nutritious than the stalks.**

6. Load up on vegetables, fruits, and salads. Limit the added fat by *asking for dressing and sauces on the side.*
7. Choose "clean" food. Instead of frying—broil, bake, grill, or poach your foods. Serve without adding fat-laden sauces. (Lemon does wonders.)
8. Limit your animal protein to a portion the size of a deck of cards (about 4 ounces). Eat such protein no more than twice a day.
9. Try to have at least 2 to 3 vegetarian days a week. Select from hearty soups, salads, vegetables, pastas, whole grain products, nonfat milk, yogurt, and fruit.

> **"After dinner sit a while, and after supper walk a mile."**
> **—English saying**

10. Drink a 6- to 8-ounce glass of water *before* each meal with a total of 6 to 8 glasses per day. (Coffee, tea, and cola drinks do not count.)
11. Exercise regularly. Start with a 15-minute walk each day and try to build to 30 to 45 minutes (about 3 miles), 5 days a week. **Or use a pedometer and try to take 10,000 steps per day.**

12. If you can lose 7 to 10 pounds, you will lower your cholesterol level, lower your blood pressure, lower your blood sugar level, and reduce your risk of diabetes, and you most certainly will feel better.

---

**Remember, the journey of a thousand miles begins with the first step.**

---

### Fat and Calories In = Pounds On

Some people count fat grams, some count calories, some count both, and **some don't count.** However, what really counts is your resulting good health. Food choices in both restaurant or take-out foods and supermarket foods have many surprising alternatives. One suggestion—try taking home half of what you order in a Chinese, Italian, or Mexican restaurant for tomorrow's lunch. Another suggestion—consider the alternative choices below:

### Consider the Alternatives ...

| Restaurant First Choice | Fat Grams | Calories | Healthier Choice | Fat Grams | Calories |
|---|---|---|---|---|---|
| Kung Pao chicken w/rice (1 order) | 76 | 1,620 | Shrimp or scallops w/ garlic sauce, snow peas, & steamed rice (1/2 order) | 14 | 470 |
| Chicken burrito w/rice, beans, sour cream, & guacamole (1 order) | 68 | 1,530 | Chicken fajitas w/rice or fat-free beans (1/2 order) | 22 | 720 |
| Pasta w/meatballs (3½ cups) | 39 | 1,155 | Pasta marinara (3½ cups) | 17 | 850 |
| | | | ½ order (1¾ cups) | 8 | 425 |
| Porterhouse steak (20 oz.) | 82 | 1,100 | Sirloin steak (12 oz.) | 18 | 410 |
| Pepperoni pizza (2 slices) | 34 | 700 | Veggie pizza, thin crust, no cheese (2 slices) | 18 | 350 |
| Tuna salad sandwich w/mayo (11 oz.) | 56 | 835 | Turkey sandwich w/mustard on whole wheat or rye bread (9 oz.) | 6 | 370 |
| Baked potato w/ bacon, butter, sour cream & cheese | 31 | 620 | Baked potato w/1 tb. light sour cream & chives | 3 | 310 |

| Restaurant First Choice | Fat Grams | Calories | Healthier Choice | Fat Grams | Calories |
|---|---|---|---|---|---|
| Ham & cheese omelet (3 eggs) | 39 | 510 | Egg white or egg substitute omelette (3 eggs) | 8 | 195 |
| Grilled cheese sandwich (5 oz.) | 33 | 510 | Veggie cheese substitute sandwich (6 oz.) | 9 | 270 |
| Movie popcorn w/butter (small cup) | 50 | 630 | Movie popcorn w/o butter (small cup) | 27 | 400 |
| Cheese Danish or blueberry muffin | 22 | 630 | Whole wheat English muffin with sugar-free jam | 2 | 140 |
| Fried chicken breast w/skin (5 oz.) | 24 | 400 | Roast chicken breast w/o skin (4 oz.) | 4 | 170 |

---

**The color of egg yolks depends on what the chicken is fed.**

---

### Decisions! Decisions! Decisions!

Try these lower-fat, healthier food choices:

| | INSTEAD OF THIS | TRY THIS |
|---|---|---|
| Beverages | 1 cup whole milk | 1 cup 1% fat or skim milk |
| | 1 chocolate milkshake | 1 cup cocoa prepared with skim milk or water |
| | 1 cup coffee with 1 tb. cream | 1 cup coffee with 1% fat milk |
| Dressing | ¼ cup sour cream | ¼ cup nonfat plain yogurt or ¼ cup nonfat sour cream |
| | ¼ cup mayonnaise | ¼ cup light or nonfat mayonnaise |
| | 2 tb. salad dressing | 1 tb. balsamic or flavored vinegar or lemon juice |
| Breakfasts | 3-egg cheese omelet | ½ cup Egg Beaters vegetable omelet or 3-egg-white omelet |
| | 2 7-inch waffles w/butter & syrup | 4 4-inch pancakes w/sugar-free jam or fresh fruit |

|  | INSTEAD OF THIS | TRY THIS |
|---|---|---|
|  | Croissant & 1 cup granola w/coconut | Water bagel & 1 cup wheat or bran flakes |
| Sandwiches | Club | Turkey |
|  | Tuna salad or chicken salad w/mayo | Chicken breast or fish w/o skin, grilled |
|  | Bologna | Lean roast beef or ham |
|  | Cheeseburger | 1/4 lb. plain lean hamburger, turkey burger, or veggie burger |
|  | 1/4 lb. regular ground sirloin | 1/4 lb. ground turkey breast |
| Soups | 1 cup New England clam chowder | 1 cup Manhattan clam chowder |
|  | 1 cup French onion soup with cheese | 1 cup vegetarian split pea soup |
|  | 1 cup cream of tomato soup | 1 cup gazpacho |
|  | 1 cup cream of chicken soup | 1 cup chicken gumbo |
| Meat, fish, poultry | 3½ oz. chicken thigh or wing w/skin | 3 oz. chicken breast or drumstick, broiled or roasted, w/o skin |
|  | Pork chop or ribs | 3 oz. pork tenderloin |
|  | Turkey thigh | Turkey drumstick, w/o skin |
|  | 3½ oz. canned tuna in oil | 3½ oz. canned tuna in water or 3½ oz. canned salmon |
|  | 3½ oz. breaded, fried fish | 3 oz. grilled, broiled, or poached fish |
|  | 3½ oz. fried shrimp w/tartar sauce | 3 oz. boiled shrimp w/cocktail sauce |
|  | 3½ oz. duck, roasted, no skin | 3 oz. chicken, roasted, no skin |
|  | Rack of lamb | Leg of lamb |
| Fast foods | Beef burrito | Baked vegetarian burrito or soft chicken or fish taco |
|  | Double burger with cheese | 1/4 pound burger or grilled chicken breast with soft bun |
|  | Chocolate malt | Low-fat chocolate milk |
|  | Fried onion rings | Baked potato |
|  | Hot cakes w/butter & syrup | English muffin w/jam |
|  | Danish | Fat-free muffin |
| Snacks | 1 oz. potato chips | 1 oz. pretzels or baked chips |
|  | 1 cup popcorn, popped in oil | 1 cup air-popped popcorn |
|  | 1 oz. milk chocolate | 1 oz. dark chocolate |
|  | 1 oz. peanuts | 2 cups air-popped popcorn |

|              | INSTEAD OF THIS | TRY THIS |
|--------------|------------------|----------|
| Desserts | 1 slice pecan pie | 1 slice apple pie (1 crust) |
| | Chocolate cake w/icing | Angel food cake w/berries |
| | 2 chocolate chip cookies | 2 vanilla wafers or fig bars |
| | 1 cup ice cream | 1 cup nonfat ice cream, frozen yogurt, or sorbet |
| Miscellaneous | 1 slice pepperoni pizza | 1 slice thin-crust vegetarian pizza |
| | 1 glazed doughnut | 1 whole wheat bagel (scooped if you like) |
| | 1 tb. butter or stick margarine | 1 tb. light tub margarine (0 trans fat) or nonfat whipped cream cheese |
| | 1 corn muffin | 1 whole wheat English muffin |
| | 1 tb. mayonnaise | 1 tb. mustard or nonfat mayonnaise |
| | 1 tb. stick margarine | 1 tb. light tub margarine |
| | 1 oz. brown gravy | 1 oz. au jus gravy |
| | 1 whole artichoke w/hollandaise sauce | 1 whole artichoke w/lemon or balsamic vinegar |
| | 1 oz. cheddar cheese | 1 oz. low-fat or nonfat cheddar cheese |
| | 1 oz. regular cream cheese | 1 oz. light or fat-free cream cheese |
| | ½ cup whole-milk cottage cheese | ½ cup nonfat cottage cheese |
| | 1 6-oz. baked potato w/butter & sour cream | 1 6-oz. baked sweet potato |
| | ½ cup hash browns | ½ baked or boiled potato |
| | 1 Snickers bar | 1 Tootsie Roll |
| | 1 oz. Hershey's Kisses | 1 oz. jelly beans |

Using low-fat and nonfat dairy products is a quick and easy way to lower your fat intake.

## Avoid Portion Distortion

Nutritionists have known for years that most people have no idea how much they eat. A **serving** is the standard amount of food listed on a label; a **portion** is the amount you choose to put on your plate.

> **"To lengthen thy life, lessen thy meals."—Benjamin Franklin.**

## What Counts As a Serving?

### Bread, Cereal, Rice, & Pasta (a cupped handful)

| | | |
|---|---|---|
| I slice of bread | I oz. ready-to-eat cereal | ½ cup cooked cereal, rice, or pasta |

### Vegetables (a closed fist or a tennis ball)

| | | |
|---|---|---|
| I cup raw, leafy vegetables | ½ cup cooked or chopped raw vegetables | ¾ cup sodium-reduced vegetable juice |

### Fruit (a closed fist or a tennis ball)

| | | |
|---|---|---|
| I medium apple, orange, or pear, or ½ banana | ½ cup chopped cooked or canned fruit | ¾ cup chopped fresh fruit |

### Milk, Yogurt, and Cheese

| | | |
|---|---|---|
| 8 oz. milk or yogurt (choose nonfat or low-fat) | I½ oz. natural cheese (approx. size: 3 dice) | 2 oz. processed cheese (approx. size: 4 dice) |

### Meat, Poultry, Fish, Dry Beans, Tofu, Eggs, & Nuts (an open palm or a deck of cards)

| | | |
|---|---|---|
| 3–4 oz. cooked lean meat, poultry, fish, or seafood | 2 tb. peanut butter equal I oz. lean meat | a handful of nuts, ½ cup cooked dry beans, or I egg |

## Knowledge Is Power in Preventive Nutrition

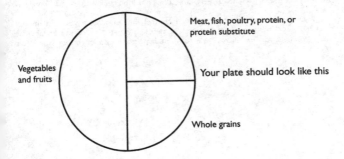

Meat, fish, poultry, protein, or protein substitute

Vegetables and fruits

Your plate should look like this

Whole grains

# In Defense of the New Food Pyramid

The new food guide pyramid, My Pyramid, is designed to carry the message of the FDA's 2005 dietary guidelines, based on the most current nutritional science. The key information is:

- Eat more whole grains, fruits, and vegetables, and nonfat or low-fat dairy products.
- Eat fewer foods that contain saturated or trans fat.
- Limit added sugar. Aim for no more than 32 grams per day.
- As previously suggested, limit cholesterol to no more than 100 milligrams per day.
- Limit added salt and alcohol.
- Last but certainly important: Be physically active every day.

My Pyramid uses a comprehensive food guide in an interactive Web site (www.mypyramid.gov). Search out a food pattern that suits your needs. There is also a special pyramid designed for children with an interactive game that helps them understand more about healthy eating. If you have specific health problems, such as obesity, diabetes, hypertension, or heart disease, seek out professional help.

This food plan is not my ideal conception of what you should eat to enjoy optimum health. However, at this time, it's the best the FDA has to offer. The most important thing is that the FDA is now addressing the urgency of **good nutrition for all**.

Most people do not follow its advice: 45% of people over the age of 2 are eating the minimum suggested serving of vegetables a day; only 28% are getting two servings of fruit; and 16% of adult women consume the daily recommended servings of dairy (3 cups or the equivalent daily). In the meantime, more than half the calories we consume are added fats—and we eat nearly triple the amount of added sugars. Unfortunately, **the pyramid does not indicate how big a serving really is**.

"All this pyramid was meant to do was illustrate variety, proportions and above all, moderation," states Jeanne Goldberg, director of nutrition communication at Tufts University.

If you get portions and calories under control with adequate physical activity, eat 5 or more servings of fruits and vegetables daily, and whole grain cereals and low-fat dairy products, you are on your way to maintaining not only a longer but a healthier life.

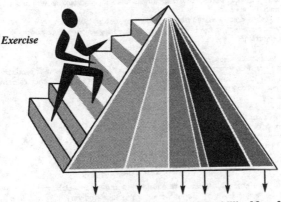

**Food Guide Pyramid**
**Developed by the U.S. Department of Agriculture and**
**Department of Health & Human Services**

*Exercise*

*Grains   Veggies   Fruits   Oils   Milk   Meat & Beans*

## Exercise

Be physically active and reduce sedentary activities.

Get 30 minutes of exercise most days of the week or 10,000 steps per day using a pedometer.

For sustaining weight loss, get 60 minutes a day of physical activity.

Children and teenagers should be physically active for 60 minutes every day.

## Grains

Eat 6 ounces a day—make half of your grains whole.

Eat at least 3 ounces of whole grain cereals, breads, crackers, rice, or pasta every day.

1 ounce is about 1 slice of bread, about 1 cup of breakfast cereal, or ½ cup of cooked rice, cereal, or pasta.

## Vegetables

Eat 2½ cups a day—vary your veggies.

Eat more dark green veggies such as broccoli, spinach, romaine, and other dark leafy greens.

Eat more orange vegetables such as carrots and sweet potatoes.

Eat more dried beans and peas, such as pinto beans, kidney beans, and lentils.

## Fruits

Eat 2 cups a day—focus on fruits.

Eat a variety of fruit.

Choose fresh, frozen, canned in natural juice, or limited dried fruit.

Go easy on fruit juices.

### Oils

In limited amounts, use olive oil, canola oil, and trans fat–free margarine.

Make most of your fat sources from fish, nuts, and vegetable oils.

Avoid solid fats such as butter, stick margarine, shortening, and lard, as well as foods that contain these.

Check the label to keep saturated fats, trans fats, and sodium low.

Choose food and beverages low in added sugars. Added sugars contribute calories with few, if any, nutrients.

### Milk

Consume 3 cups a day—get your calcium-rich foods.

Go low-fat or fat-free when you choose milk, yogurt, cheese, and other milk products.

If you don't or can't consume milk, choose lactose-free products or other calcium sources such as soy products, fortified foods, and beverages.

### Meat & Beans

Eat 5½ ounces a day—go lean with your protein.

Choose low-fat or lean meats and poultry.

Bake it, broil it, or grill it.

Vary your protein sources—choose more fish (see page xxi), dried beans, split peas, nuts, and seeds.

### The Bottom Line

We used to think that all calories were equally responsible for weight gain. We now know that the various kinds of calories we eat are metabolized very differently in our bodies.

We used to think that blood cholesterol levels were raised by dietary cholesterol alone. **We now know that foods high in saturated fat and trans-fatty acids raise cholesterol levels more than dietary cholesterol itself does.**

We used to think that high blood pressure was caused by genetics alone. We now know that lifestyle changes, such as reducing sodium consumption to less than 1,500 milligrams per day, losing excess weight, limiting alcohol consumption to no more than 1 drink per day, routine exercise, and other lifestyle changes, such as eating 8 to 10 servings a day of veggies and fruits, can lower or prevent high blood pressure.

**When it comes to your health, everyone else seems to know what's best for you, and "experts" are quick to tell you what habits to change. There are the high-protein and low-protein diets; high-carbohydrate and low-carbohydrate diets; the pasta diet; the raw food diet; the rice and fruit diet, and, depending on when you read this book, endless new suggestions. Let your common sense prevail about what and *how much* you eat.**

As consumers, we get tired of the barrage of new information. The only sensible re-course that we have is to try to understand and apply the most current information available—in moderation. The more we learn about nutrition, the more we realize we have to learn. We now know that it is not only the total fat but the kind of fat you eat that is important. Limit those trans fats and saturated fats.

Today's children are overfed and underexercised, resulting in childhood obesity that has reached epidemic proportions. Unless we reverse this trend, our children may have *shorter* rather than *longer* life expectancies than we now pursue as adults.

My strong beliefs in the fundamentals of a healthful diet are unchanged. Eat fewer foods that contain saturated fat or trans fat. Limit added sugar, cholesterol, salt, and alcoholic beverages. Include fruits, vegetables, and whole grains—foods that you know contain the nutrients that you need to keep you healthy. In a word, watch what you eat and *how much you eat*.

This book is for people who love to eat but are still concerned about the impact food has on their health. This extraordinary little counter and **food digest** lists thousands of foods from appetizers to desserts, soups to salads, main dishes to snacks, and even covers dining out and fast foods. It's small enough to fit in your purse or pocket, to consult whether in a supermarket, fast-food chain, or restaurant. It's all here for your convenience and good health. My best wishes for your good health and longevity. Enjoy.

H.R.

Note: Recipes for all entries that are preceded by an asterisk (*) can be found in *Harriet Roth's Cholesterol-Control Cookbook* (Plume, $18.00).

> Sooner or later, we all sit down to a banquet of consequences.
> —Robert Louis Stevenson.

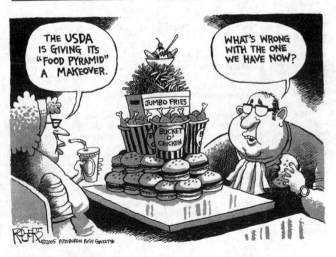

Rob Rogers: © *The Pittsburgh Post-Gazette*/Dist. by United Feature Syndicate, Inc.

**Blood glucose** is a simple form of sugar that acts as the body's fuel. It results when foods are broken down in the process of digestion. Glucose is then carried by the blood to the cells.

**Body mass index (BMI)** measures your height in relationship to your weight.

**Calories** represent the amount of energy provided by food. Carbohydrates, protein, and fat are the primary sources of calories in the diet, but alcohol also provides calories. If all calories aren't used, they may be stored as fat.

**Carbohydrates** are one of three major sources of calories in the diet. Carbohydrates come primarily from sugar (simple carbohydrates) and starch (complex carbohydrates, found in bread, pasta, and beans).

**Cholesterol** is a waxy, fatlike substance used by the body to build cell walls and make certain vitamins and hormones. The liver produces enough cholesterol for the body, but we also get cholesterol when we eat animal products. Eating too much cholesterol, saturated fat, and trans fat can cause the blood cholesterol to rise and collect along the inside walls of blood vessels. This is a risk factor for heart attack and stroke.

**C-reactive protein (CRP)** is a test that measures the concentration of a protein in the blood that indicates inflammation. This test is a powerful predictor of cardiovascular disease and type 2 diabetes.

**DASH diet** is an eating plan that helps control blood pressure and may also improve cholesterol level. It is rich in vegetables and fruits and low in saturated fat, trans fat, and cholesterol.

**Diabetes** is a disease in which the body cannot produce insulin or cannot use insulin to its full potential.
> **Type 1 diabetes** is a form of diabetes that tends to develop before age 30 but may occur at any age. It is caused by an immune system attack on the insulin-producing beta cells of the pancreas. People who have type 1 diabetes must take insulin to survive.
> **Type 2 diabetes** usually occurs in people over 40 years of age but is increasingly being diagnosed in younger people, especially among minorities. Most people who develop type 2 diabetes are insulin resistant. Some simply cannot produce enough insulin to meet their bodies' needs. Some people with type 2 diabetes control the disease with diet and exercise, but most must also take oral medications or insulin.

**Fats** are the most concentrated source of calories in the diet. Saturated fats are found primarily in animal products. Unsaturated fats come mainly from plants. Excess intake of fat, especially saturated fat and trans-fatty acids, can cause elevated blood cholesterol, increasing the risk of heart disease and stroke.

**Fiber** is the part of a plant that the body can't digest, such as fruit and vegetable pulp and skins. Fiber aids in the normal functioning of the digestive system, specifically the intestinal tract.

**Glycemic index (GI)** is a system of ranking foods that contain carbohydrates according to how much they raise blood sugar. Some carbohydrates raise the blood sugar level more than others do. Glycemic index values range from 0 to 100. Foods with lower values have less of an effect on blood glucose than do foods with higher values.

**Heart disease** is a condition in which the heart cannot efficiently pump blood. Coronary artery disease is the most common form of heart disease. It occurs when the arteries that nourish the heart muscle narrow or become blocked.

**High-density lipoprotein (HDL)** is sometimes referred to as the *good cholesterol*. A healthy level is 50 mg/dL or higher.

**Homocysteine** is an amino acid. High blood levels of homocysteine are associated with a higher risk of heart disease, stroke, and peripheral vascular disease. People with diabetes need to watch their homocysteine levels very carefully.

**Hyperglycemia** is a condition in which blood sugar levels are too high. Symptoms include frequent urination, increased thirst, and weight loss.

**Hypoglycemia** is a condition in which blood sugar levels drop too low. Symptoms include moodiness, numbness, confusion, and shakiness or dizziness.

**Low-density lipoprotein (LDL)** is referred to as the *bad cholesterol*. Desirable numbers are under 100 milligrams per deciliter.

**My Pyramid** is a graphic designed to express the message of the FDA's 2005 dietary guidelines, which are based on the latest nutritional science.

**Nutrigenomics** is a promising new study that will customize your food needs to your genes and metabolism. It will provide an individualized dietary roadmap. (It is nothing like the traditional food pyramid, one-size-fits-all approach.)

**Obesity** is an abnormal and excessive amount of body fat. Obesity is considered a chronic illness. It is on the rise and is a risk factor for type 2 diabetes.

**Protein** is one of three major sources of calories in the diet. Protein provides the body with material for building blood cells, body tissue, hormones, and other important substances. It is found in meats, eggs, milk, and certain vegetables and starches.

# NUTRITIONAL ANALYSIS

In January 2006, the Food and Drug Administration began requiring that package labels list trans fat contents. Trans fats are artificial fats made when hydrogen gas reacts with liquid oils, resulting in a partially hydrogenated oil. The result is a stiffer fat, like the fat found in Crisco and stick margarine. Trans fats are also called hydrogenated or partially hydrogenated fats.

Ruminants—animals such as domestic cattle, buffalo, deer, and giraffe—chew their cuds, and as a result, seem to produce some trans fat. However, veal, lamb, and pork contain little or no discernible trans fat.

Trans fats cause a higher risk of heart disease than saturated fats. *Trans fats not only raise the bad cholesterol levels (LDL), but also lower the good cholesterol (HDL).*

Current research seems to point toward a daily recommended amount of trans fat of *no more than 5.0 mg.* This information helps protect us against heart disease.

### ZERO DOES NOT ALWAYS = 0 IT WILL ADD UP IN TIME!

> **Caution**—Legally processed foods may have **up to 0.5 milligrams of trans fat** listed in a serving and **still list it on the label as "0 mg."** trans fat. Therefore, if you use a spread or crackers listed as containing 0 mg of trans fat, you could be consuming larger amounts of trans fat. As a consumer, you can protect yourself only by using products labeled **"contains no trans fat"** or whose ingredient list does not include shortening, partially hydrogenated vegetable oil, or hydrogenated oil.

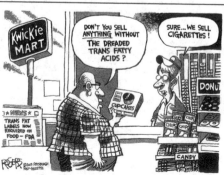

Rob Rogers: © *The Pittsburgh Post-Gazette*/Dist. by United Feature Syndicate, Inc.

| Item | SERVING | CAL-ORIES | FAT GRAMS | SAT. FAT GRAMS | TRANS FAT GRAMS | CARB. GRAMS | SUGAR GRAMS |
|---|---|---|---|---|---|---|---|
| **BEVERAGES** | | | | | | | |
| **Alcoholic** | | | | | | | |
| Ale, brown, bottled | 12 fl.oz. | 169 | 0.0 | 0.0 | 0.0 | 14.0 | n/a |
| Beer | | | | | | | |
| Regular | 12 fl.oz. | 139 | 0.0 | 0.0 | 0.0 | 10.8 | 0.0 |
| Light | 12 fl.oz. | 103 | 0.0 | 0.0 | 0.0 | 5.2 | 0.3 |
| Bloody Mary | 6 fl.oz. | 46 | 0.0 | 0.0 | 0.0 | 7.5 | 4.6 |
| Champagne | 6 fl.oz. | 128 | 0.0 | 0.0 | 0.0 | 3.0 | 3.0 |
| Daiquiri, frozen | 6 fl.oz. | 316 | 0.2 | 0.0 | 0.0 | 11.6 | 11.6 |
| Gin | | | | | | | |
| 80 proof | 1.5 fl.oz. | 96 | 0.0 | 0.0 | 0.0 | 0.0 | 0.0 |
| 86 proof | 1.5 fl.oz. | 104 | 0.0 | 0.0 | 0.0 | 0.0 | 0.0 |
| 90 proof | 1.5 fl.oz. | 112 | 0.0 | 0.0 | 0.0 | 0.0 | 0.0 |
| 100 proof | 1.5 fl.oz. | 123 | 0.0 | 0.0 | 0.0 | 0.0 | 0.0 |
| Margarita | 6 fl.oz. | 375 | 0.2 | 0.0 | 0.0 | 23.8 | 22.2 |
| Pina colada | 6 fl.oz. | 327 | 3.6 | 3.1 | 0.0 | 42.6 | n/a |
| Rum | | | | | | | |
| 80 proof | 1.5 fl.oz. | 96 | 0.0 | 0.0 | 0.0 | 0.0 | 0.0 |
| 86 proof | 1.5 fl.oz. | 106 | 0.0 | 0.0 | 0.0 | 0.0 | 0.0 |
| 90 proof | 1.5 fl.oz. | 112 | 0.0 | 0.0 | 0.0 | 0.0 | 0.0 |
| 100 proof | 1.5 fl.oz. | 125 | 0.0 | 0.0 | 0.0 | 0.0 | 0.0 |
| Sherry, dry | 6 fl.oz. | 123 | 0.0 | 0.0 | 0.0 | 2.5 | n/a |
| Tequila sunrise | 6 fl.oz. | 205 | 0.2 | 0.0 | 0.0 | 21.1 | n/a |
| Vodka | | | | | | | |
| 80 proof | 1.5 fl.oz. | 96 | 0.0 | 0.0 | 0.0 | 0.0 | 0.0 |
| 86 proof | 1.5 fl.oz. | 104 | 0.0 | 0.0 | 0.0 | 0.0 | 0.0 |
| 90 proof | 1.5 fl.oz. | 110 | 0.0 | 0.0 | 0.0 | 0.0 | 0.0 |
| 100 proof | 1.5 fl.oz. | 123 | 0.0 | 0.0 | 0.0 | 0.0 | 0.0 |
| Whiskey | | | | | | | |
| 80 proof | 1.5 fl.oz. | 98 | 0.0 | 0.0 | 0.0 | 0.0 | 0.0 |
| 86 proof | 1.5 fl.oz. | 104 | 0.0 | 0.0 | 0.0 | 0.0 | n/a |
| 90 proof | 1.5 fl.oz. | 110 | 0.0 | 0.0 | 0.0 | 0.0 | 0.0 |
| 100 Proof | 1.5 fl.oz. | 133 | 0.0 | 0.0 | 0.0 | 0.0 | 0.0 |
| Wine | | | | | | | |
| Cooler/spritzer | 6 fl.oz. | 71 | 0.0 | 0.0 | 0.0 | 1.4 | n/a |
| Dessert, Dry | 6 fl.oz. | 269 | 0.0 | 0.0 | 0.0 | 20.7 | 1.9 |
| Sweet | 6 fl.oz. | 283 | 0.0 | 0.0 | 0.0 | 24.2 | 13.8 |
| Muscatel | 6 fl.oz. | 255 | 0.0 | 0.0 | 0.0 | 15.0 | 15.0 |
| Red | 6 fl.oz. | 127 | 0.0 | 0.0 | 0.0 | 3.0 | n/a |
| White, dry | 6 fl.oz. | 122 | 0.0 | 0.0 | 0.0 | 1.5 | 1.5 |
| **Nonalcoholic** | | | | | | | |
| ■ Beer, O'Doul's | 12 fl.oz. | 70 | 0.0 | 0.0 | 0.0 | 15.0 | n/a |
| Coffee | | | | | | | |
| ■ Brewed, regular | 6 fl.oz. | 2 | 0.0 | 0.0 | 0.0 | 0.0 | 0.0 |

■ Contains less than 20% fat
n/a Not available

| Item | SERVING | CAL-ORIES | FAT GRAMS | SAT. FAT GRAMS | TRANS FAT GRAMS | CARB. GRAMS | SUGAR GRAMS |
|---|---|---|---|---|---|---|---|
| ■ Instant | 6 fl.oz. | 4 | 0.0 | 0.0 | 0.0 | 0.6 | 0.0 |
| Flavored, General Foods | | | | | | | |
| Café Francais | 6 fl.oz. | 41 | 2.4 | 0.7 | 0.0 | 4.8 | 2.7 |
| Café Vienna | 6 fl.oz. | 53 | 1.9 | 0.4 | 0.0 | 8.3 | 6.8 |
| French Vanilla Café | 6 fl.oz. | 41 | 1.7 | 0.3 | 0.0 | 6.8 | 4.8 |
| ■ French Vanilla Café, fat & sugar free | 6 fl.oz. | 19 | 0.0 | 0.0 | 0.0 | 3.8 | 0.0 |
| Swiss Mocha | 6 fl.oz. | 45 | 1.5 | 0.4 | 0.0 | 6.8 | 5.3 |
| ■ Swiss Mocha, fat & sugar free | 6 fl.oz. | 19 | 0.0 | 0.0 | 0.0 | 3.8 | 0.0 |
| Starbucks | | | | | | | |
| Cappuccino, w/whole milk, tall | 12 fl.oz. | 120 | 6.0 | 4.0 | n/a | 10.0 | 9.0 |
| ■ w/nonfat milk, tall | 12 fl.oz. | 80 | 0.0 | 0.0 | 0.0 | 11.0 | 9.0 |
| ■ Espresso | 3 fl.oz. | 15 | 0.0 | 0.0 | 0.0 | 3.0 | 0.0 |
| ■ Frappuccino, mocha, tall, w/o whipped cream | 12 fl. oz. | 220 | 3.0 | 1.5 | 0.0 | 44 | 36.0 |
| ■ Frappuccino, mocha, light, tall | 12 fl.oz. | 140 | 1.5 | 0.0 | 0.0 | 28 | 19.0 |
| Latte, w/whole milk, tall | 12 fl.oz. | 200 | 11.0 | 7.0 | 0.0 | 11.3 | 10.7 |
| ■ Latte, w/nonfat milk, tall | 12 fl.oz. | 120 | 0.0 | 0.0 | 0.0 | 18 | 16.0 |
| Latte, iced, w/whole milk, tall | 12 fl.oz. | 120 | 6.0 | 4.0 | 0.0 | 10.0 | 9.0 |
| ■ Latte, iced, w/nonfat milk, tall | 12 fl.oz. | 70 | 0.0 | 0.0 | 0.0 | 11.0 | 7.0 |
| ■ Crystal Light | 8 fl.oz. | 5 | 0.0 | 0.0 | 0.0 | 0.0 | 0.0 |
| ■ Classic Orange, bottle | 8 fl.oz. | 0 | 0.0 | 0.0 | 0.0 | 0.0 | 0.0 |
| ■ Dr. Pepper | 12 fl.oz. | 150 | 0.0 | 0.0 | 0.0 | 37.0 | 37.0 |
| ■ Fresca | 12 fl.oz. | 4 | 0.0 | 0.0 | 0.0 | 0.3 | 0.3 |
| ■ Fruit punch, canned | 8 fl.oz. | 117 | 0.0 | 0.0 | 0.0 | 29.7 | 28.0 |
| ■ Gatorade, Citrus Cooler | 8 fl.oz. | 60 | 0.0 | 0.0 | 0.0 | 15.2 | n/a |
| ■ Grape drink, Hi-C, 10% juice, box | 1 each | 130 | 0.0 | 0.0 | 0.0 | 34.0 | 33.0 |
| Juice | | | | | | | |
| ■ Apple | ½ cup | 55 | 0.0 | 0.0 | 0.0 | 14.5 | 14.5 |
| ■ Apple/cranberry | ½ cup | 70 | 0.0 | 0.0 | 0.0 | 17.0 | 16.4 |
| ■ Apple, sparkling, Martinelli's | 8 fl.oz. | 140 | 0.0 | 0.0 | 0.0 | 35.0 | 31.0 |
| ■ Carrot, Odwalla | 8 fl.oz. | 70 | 0.0 | 0.0 | 0.0 | 15.0 | 13.0 |
| ■ Clam | 5 fl.oz. | 3 | 0.0 | 0.0 | 0.0 | 0.2 | 0.0 |
| ■ Cranberry, Ocean Spray | 8 fl.oz. | 130 | 0.0 | 0.0 | 0.0 | 33.0 | 33.0 |
| ■ Grape, Welch's | 8 fl.oz. | 170 | 0.0 | 0.0 | 0.0 | 42.0 | 40.0 |
| ■ Light | 8 fl.oz. | 70 | 0.0 | 0.0 | 0.0 | 18.0 | 17.0 |
| ■ Grapefruit, canned, unsweetened | ½ cup | 47 | 0.1 | 0.0 | 0.0 | 11.1 | 10.9 |
| Sweetened | ½ cup | 58 | 0.1 | 0.0 | 0.0 | 13.9 | 13.8 |
| ■ Orange, fresh | ½ cup | 56 | 0.3 | 0.0 | 0.0 | 12.9 | 10.4 |
| ■ Orange/pineapple | ½ cup | 55 | 0.0 | 0.0 | 0.0 | 13.5 | 12.0 |
| ■ Passionfruit, Fizzy Lizzy | 12 fl.oz. | 150 | 0.0 | 0.0 | 0.0 | 33.0 | 30.0 |
| ■ Pineapple, unsweetened | ½ cup | 70 | 0.1 | 0.0 | 0.0 | 17.2 | 17.0 |
| ■ Pineapple/grapefruit | ½ cup | 59 | 0.1 | 0.0 | 0.0 | 14.5 | 14.4 |
| ■ Pomegranate, Pom Wonderful | 8 fl.oz. | 140 | 0.0 | 0.0 | 0.0 | 35.0 | 34.0 |
| ■ Prune | ½ cup | 85 | 0.0 | 0.0 | 0.0 | 21.0 | 8.0 |

■ Contains less than 20% fat
n/a Not available

| Item | SERVING | CALORIES | FAT GRAMS | SAT. FAT GRAMS | TRANS FAT GRAMS | CARB. GRAMS | SUGAR GRAMS |
|---|---|---|---|---|---|---|---|
| Tomato | | | | | | | |
| ■ Campbell | ½ cup | 25 | 0.0 | 0.0 | 0.0 | 6.0 | 4.0 |
| ■ Low sodium | 8 fl.oz. | 50 | 0.0 | 0.0 | 0.0 | 10.0 | 7.0 |
| ■ V8 | ½ cup | 25 | 0.0 | 0.0 | 0.0 | 5.0 | 3.5 |
| ■ Low sodium | ½ cup | 25 | 0.0 | 0.0 | 0.0 | 5.5 | 4.0 |
| ■ Kool-Aid, cherry | 1 cup | 60 | 0.0 | 0.0 | 0.0 | 16.0 | 16.0 |
| Lemonade | | | | | | | |
| ■ Country Time, sugar sweetened, mix | 1 cup | 70 | 0.0 | 0.0 | 0.0 | 17.0 | 17.0 |
| ■ Sugar free, low cal, mix | 1 cup | 5 | 0.0 | 0.0 | 0.0 | 0.0 | 0.0 |
| ■ Pink, sugar sweetened, mix | 1 cup | 70 | 0.0 | 0.0 | 0.0 | 17.0 | 17.0 |
| ■ Sugar free, low cal, prepared | 1 cup | 5 | 0.0 | 0.0 | 0.0 | 0.0 | 0.0 |
| ■ From frozen concentrate w/water | 1 cup | 131 | 0.2 | 0.0 | 0.0 | 34.1 | 32.6 |
| ■ Limeade | 1 cup | 104 | 0.0 | 0.0 | 0.0 | 26.1 | 22.2 |
| Meal replacements/supplements | | | | | | | |
| Ensure, chocolate | 1 can | 250 | 6.0 | 0.5 | 0.0 | 40.0 | 18.0 |
| Nutrifull, Vitasoy, Strawberry | 1 bottle | 200 | 1.0 | 0.0 | 0.0 | 39.0 | 31.0 |
| Slimfast milk chocolate | 1 can | 180 | 5.0 | 1.0 | 0.0 | 24.0 | 17.0 |
| Milk (see Dairy & Dairy Products, milk) | | | | | | | |
| Nectar, canned | | | | | | | |
| ■ Apricot | ½ cup | 70 | 0.1 | 0.0 | 0.0 | 18.1 | n/a |
| ■ Peach | ½ cup | 67 | 0.0 | 0.0 | 0.0 | 17.3 | n/a |
| ■ Seltzer | 10 fl.oz. | 0 | 0.0 | 0.0 | 0.0 | 0.0 | 0.0 |
| Smoothie | | | | | | | |
| ■ Banana Berry, Jamba Juice | 24 fl.oz. | 470 | 1.5 | 0.5 | 0.0 | 112.0 | 100.0 |
| ■ Mango Tango, Odwalla | 8 fl.oz. | 150 | 1.0 | 0.5 | 0.0 | 34.0 | 30.0 |
| Soda | | | | | | | |
| ■ Club | 12 fl.oz. | 0 | 0.0 | 0.0 | 0.0 | 0.0 | 0.0 |
| ■ Coca-Cola/Coke | 12 fl.oz. | 154 | 0.0 | 0.0 | 0.0 | 40.0 | 40.0 |
| Diet | 12 fl.oz. | 2 | 0.0 | 0.0 | 0.0 | 0.1 | 0.1 |
| ■ Cream | 12 fl.oz. | 189 | 0.0 | 0.0 | 0.0 | 49.3 | 49.3 |
| ■ Ginger ale | 12 fl.oz. | 124 | 0.0 | 0.0 | 0.0 | 32.1 | 31.8 |
| ■ Grape | 12 fl.oz. | 160 | 0.0 | 0.0 | 0.0 | 41.7 | n/a |
| ■ Mountain Dew | 12 fl.oz. | 170 | 0.0 | 0.0 | 0.0 | 46.0 | 46.0 |
| ■ Orange | 12 fl.oz. | 179 | 0.0 | 0.0 | 0.0 | 45.8 | n/a |
| ■ Red Bull | 8.3 fl.oz. | 110 | 0.0 | 0.0 | 0.0 | 28.0 | 27.0 |
| ■ Sugar free | 8.3 fl.oz. | 10 | 0.0 | 0.0 | 0.0 | 3.0 | 2.0 |
| ■ Root beer | 12 fl.oz. | 152 | 0.0 | 0.0 | 0.0 | 39.2 | 39.2 |
| ■ 7 Up | 12 fl.oz. | 150 | 0.0 | 0.0 | 0.0 | 39.0 | 39.0 |
| Diet | 12 fl.oz. | 0 | 0.0 | 0.0 | 0.0 | 0.0 | 0.0 |
| ■ Sunny Delight | 8 fl.oz. | 120 | 0.0 | 0.0 | 0.0 | 29.0 | 27.0 |
| ■ Superfood, Odwalla | 8 fl.oz. | 130 | 0.5 | 0.0 | 0.0 | 30.0 | 25.0 |
| ■ Tea, black, brewed | 6 fl.oz. | 0 | 0.0 | 0.0 | 0.0 | 0.0 | 0.0 |

■ Contains less than 20% fat

n/a Not available

| Item | SERVING | CAL-ORIES | FAT GRAMS | SAT. FAT GRAMS | TRANS FAT GRAMS | CARB. GRAMS | SUGAR GRAMS |
|---|---|---|---|---|---|---|---|
| Iced | | | | | | | |
| ■ Lipton, sweetened | 1 cup | 70 | 0.0 | 0.0 | 0.0 | 18.0 | 18.0 |
| ■ Unsweetened | 1 cup | 0 | 0.0 | 0.0 | 0.0 | 0.0 | 0.0 |
| ■ Diet, w/lemon | 1 cup | 0 | 0.0 | 0.0 | 0.0 | 1.0 | 0.0 |
| ■ Tazo, w/lemon | 8 fl.oz. | 80 | 0.0 | 0.0 | 0.0 | 20.0 | 20.0 |
| Water | | | | | | | |
| ■ Propel Fitness, Tropical Citrus | 8 fl.oz. | 10 | 0.0 | 0.0 | 0.0 | 3.0 | 2.0 |
| ■ Water, tonic | 12 fl.oz. | 124 | 0.0 | 0.0 | 0.0 | 32.2 | 0.0 |

## BREADS & BREADSTUFFS

### Bagels

| Item | SERVING | CAL-ORIES | FAT GRAMS | SAT. FAT GRAMS | TRANS FAT GRAMS | CARB. GRAMS | SUGAR GRAMS |
|---|---|---|---|---|---|---|---|
| Egg | | | | | | | |
| ■ Lender's Original | 1 | 150 | 1.0 | 0.5 | 0.0 | 29.0 | 3.0 |
| ■ Big 'n Crusty | 1 | 240 | 1.5 | 0.5 | 0.0 | 49.0 | 5.0 |
| Onion | | | | | | | |
| ■ Bruegger's | 1 | 310 | 2.0 | 0.0 | 0.0 | 62.0 | 8.0 |
| ■ Lender's Original | 1 | 140 | 0.5 | 0.0 | 0.0 | 30.0 | 2.0 |
| ■ Big 'n Crusty | 1 | 240 | 1.0 | 0.5 | 0.0 | 49.0 | 4.0 |
| ■ Sara Lee | 1 | 250 | 1.0 | 0.0 | 0.0 | 51.0 | 5.0 |
| ■ Thomas', onion | 1 | 290 | 2.0 | 0.5 | 0.0 | 57.0 | 7.0 |
| Plain | | | | | | | |
| ■ Bruegger's | 1 | 300 | 2.0 | 0.0 | 0.0 | 61.0 | 0.0 |
| ■ Dunkin' Donuts | 1 | 320 | 2.5 | 0.5 | 0.0 | 62.0 | 4.0 |
| ■ Lender's Original | 1 | 140 | 0.5 | 0.0 | 0.0 | 29.0 | 2.0 |
| ■ Big 'n Crusty | 1 | 230 | 1.0 | 0.5 | 0.0 | 47.0 | 3.0 |
| ■ Sara Lee | 1 | 250 | 1.0 | 0.0 | 0.0 | 52.0 | 5.0 |
| ■ Thomas', New York style | 1 | 290 | 2.0 | 0.5 | 0.0 | 56.0 | 7.0 |
| Cinnamon raisin | | | | | | | |
| ■ Lender's Original | 1 | 150 | 1.0 | 0.0 | 0.0 | 31.0 | 6.0 |
| ■ Big 'n Crusty | 1 | 250 | 1.5 | 0.5 | n/a | 51.0 | 10.0 |
| ■ Thomas', New York style | 1 | 290 | 2.0 | 0.5 | 0.0 | 58.0 | 14.0 |
| Whole wheat | | | | | | | |
| ■ Bruegger's | 1 | 380 | 6.0 | 0.5 | 0.0 | 70.0 | 8.0 |
| ■ Sara Lee | 1 | 220 | 1.5 | 0.0 | 0.0 | 47.0 | 9.0 |
| ■ Thomas' | 1 | 250 | 2.0 | 0.0 | 0.0 | 27.0 | 3.0 |
| Bagel spreads | | | | | | | |
| Plain cream cheese, Bruegger's | 2 tb. | 90 | 8.0 | 5.0 | 0.0 | 4.0 | 1.0 |
| Smoked salmon | 2 tb. | 100 | 9.0 | 4.5 | 0.0 | 2.0 | 1.0 |
| Dunkin' Donuts | 2 tb. | 70 | 4.5 | 2.0 | 0.0 | 3.0 | 2.0 |
| Lite cream cheese | 2 oz. | 110 | 9.0 | 7.0 | 0.0 | 6.0 | 0.0 |
| Plain cream cheese | 2 oz. | 190 | 17.0 | 13.0 | 0.0 | 4.0 | 2.0 |
| Salmon cream cheese | 2 oz. | 170 | 17.0 | 11.0 | 0.0 | 2.0 | 0.0 |
| ■ Bialy | 1 | 190 | 2.3 | 0.3 | 0.0 | 36.4 | n/a |

### Biscuits

| Item | SERVING | CAL-ORIES | FAT GRAMS | SAT. FAT GRAMS | TRANS FAT GRAMS | CARB. GRAMS | SUGAR GRAMS |
|---|---|---|---|---|---|---|---|
| Gold Medal, mix | 1 | 170 | 8.0 | 3.0 | n/a | 24.0 | 1.0 |
| Perfect Portions, buttermilk | 1 | 200 | 10.0 | 3.0 | 4.5 | 25.0 | 5.0 |

| Item | SERVING | CAL-ORIES | FAT GRAMS | SAT. FAT GRAMS | TRANS FAT GRAMS | CARB. GRAMS | SUGAR GRAMS |
|---|---|---|---|---|---|---|---|
| ■ Pillsbury, country style, refrigerated dough | 1 | 50 | 0.7 | 0.0 | 0.0 | 9.7 | 1.0 |
| **Breads** | | | | | | | |
| ■ Baguette, La Brea Bakery | 1 slice | 149 | 0.0 | 0.0 | 0.0 | 31.9 | 0.0 |
| Challah bread | 1 slice | 200 | 7.0 | 1.5 | 0.0 | 29.0 | 4.0 |
| ■ Cornbread & muffin mix, Betty Crocker | 1 muffin | 160 | 1.0 | 0.0 | 0.0 | 24.0 | 6.0 |
| French | | | | | | | |
| ■ Country, Oroweat | 2 oz. | 149 | 1.5 | 0.0 | 0.0 | 28.4 | 1.5 |
| ■ Pillsbury, Crusty Loaf, low fat | 1/5 package | 150 | 2.0 | 0.5 | 0.5 | 28.0 | 3.0 |
| ■ Vienna | 1 oz. | 78 | 0.9 | 0.2 | 0.0 | 14.7 | 0.1 |
| Garlic, frozen, Mamma Bella | 2 slices | 150 | 8.0 | 3.0 | 0.0 | 16.0 | 1.0 |
| ■ Italian | 2 oz. | 154 | 2.0 | 0.5 | 0.0 | 28.4 | 0.7 |
| ■ Oatmeal, homemade | 1 slice | 73 | 1.2 | 0.2 | 0.0 | 13.1 | 2.2 |
| ■ Olive, La Brea Bakery | 1 slice | 150 | 2.0 | 0.0 | 0.0 | 28.0 | <1 |
| ■ Pita, white, 6½" | 1 | 165 | 0.7 | 0.1 | 0.0 | 33.4 | 0.8 |
| ■ Whole wheat | 1 | 154 | 0.0 | 0.0 | 0.0 | 30.0 | 0.0 |
| ■ Pumpernickel, dark, Pepperidge Farm | 1 slice | 80 | 1.0 | 0.5 | 0.0 | 15.0 | 1.0 |
| ■ Raisin cinnamon swirl, Pepperidge Farm | 1 slice | 80 | 1.5 | 0.0 | 0.0 | 14.0 | 6.0 |
| Trader Joe's | 1 slice | 80 | 0.5 | 0.0 | 0.0 | 16.0 | 6.0 |
| ■ Rye, Jewish, Oroweat | 1 slice | 80 | 1.0 | 0.0 | 0.0 | 14.0 | 1.0 |
| ■ 7 grain | 1 slice | 65 | 1.0 | 0.2 | 0.0 | 12.1 | 2.6 |
| ■ Sourdough, round, Trader Joe's | 1 slice | 150 | 0.0 | 0.0 | 0.0 | 31.0 | <1 |
| ■ Old Country | 2 oz. | 154 | 0.6 | 0.0 | 0.0 | 29.5 | 1.2 |
| ■ Spelt, Trader Joe's | 1 slice | 70 | 0.0 | 0.0 | 0.0 | 16.0 | 2.0 |
| ■ Wheat | 1 slice | 65 | 1.0 | 0.2 | 0.0 | 11.8 | 1.4 |
| ■ Country, Oroweat | 1 slice | 120 | 2.0 | 1.0 | 0.0 | 22.0 | 5.0 |
| ■ Light style, Pepperidge Farm | 1 slice | 43 | 0.3 | 0.2 | 0.0 | 9.3 | 1.0 |
| ■ Cracked Wheat | 1 slice | 80 | 1.0 | 0.0 | 0.0 | 16.0 | 1.0 |
| ■ White, Oroweat | 1 slice | 70 | 1.0 | 0.0 | 0.0 | 14.0 | 1.0 |
| ■ Pepperidge Farm | 1 slice | 65 | 1.0 | 0.3 | 0.0 | 11.5 | 1.5 |
| ■ Whole wheat | 1 slice | 69 | 1.2 | 0.3 | 0.0 | 12.9 | 5.6 |
| ■ Oroweat, 100% | 1 slice | 70 | 1.0 | 0.0 | 0.0 | 14.0 | 2.0 |
| ■ Light, 100% | 1 slice | 40 | 0.3 | 0.0 | 0.0 | 9.0 | 1.5 |
| ■ Sugar free, 100% | 1 slice | 100 | 1.5 | 0.0 | 0.0 | 18.0 | 0.0 |
| ■ Pepperidge Farm, thin sliced | 1 slice | 60 | 1.0 | 0.0 | 0.0 | 11.0 | 1.0 |
| ■ Trader Joe's | 1 slice | 70 | 1.0 | 0.0 | 0.0 | 14.0 | <1 |
| ■ Whole Foods | 1 slice | 90 | 1.5 | 0.0 | 0.0 | 18.0 | 2.0 |
| **Breads, Sweetened** | | | | | | | |
| Coffee cake, Entenmann's | 2 oz. | 200 | 9.0 | 4.5 | 0.0 | 25.0 | 12.0 |
| Sara Lee crumb | 1 piece | 190 | 8.0 | 1.5 | 0.0 | 30.0 | 18.0 |

■ Contains less than 20% fat

| Item | SERVING | CAL-ORIES | FAT GRAMS | SAT. FAT GRAMS | TRANS FAT GRAMS | CARB. GRAMS | SUGAR GRAMS |
|---|---|---|---|---|---|---|---|
| **Danish** | | | | | | | |
| Apple | 1 piece | 263 | 13.1 | 3.5 | n/a | 33.9 | 19.6 |
| Cheese, Entenmann's | 2 oz. | 220 | 12 | 5.0 | 0.0 | 27.0 | 14.0 |
| ■ Raspberry Twist, fat free, Entenmann's | 2 oz. | 220 | 11.0 | 5.0 | 0.0 | 28.0 | 15.0 |
| **Donut** | | | | | | | |
| Dunkin' Donuts | | | | | | | |
| Cake | 1 | 310 | 19.0 | 4.0 | 5.0 | 30.0 | 12.0 |
| Chocolate cake | 1 | 210 | 14.0 | 3.0 | 5.0 | 19.0 | 6.0 |
| Glazed | 1 | 160 | 7.0 | 2.0 | 5.0 | 23.0 | 5.0 |
| Entenmann's Glazed Buttermilk | 1 | 270 | 14.0 | 6.0 | 0.0 | 34 | 22 |
| Honey buns | 1 bun | 220 | 12.0 | 6.0 | 0.0 | 26.0 | 13.0 |
| Sweet rolls | | | | | | | |
| Cinnamon, w/icing, refrigerated dough, Pillsbury | 1 | 150 | 6.0 | 1.5 | 1.5 | 23.0 | 11.0 |
| Reduced fat | 1 | 140 | 3.5 | 1.0 | 1.5 | 24.0 | 10.0 |
| **Muffins** | | | | | | | |
| Plain, homemade | 1 | 169 | 6.5 | 1.2 | 0.0 | 23.6 | n/a |
| Banana Walnut, Dunkin' Donuts | 1 | 540 | 25.0 | 3.5 | 0.0 | 69.0 | 31.0 |
| ■ Blueberry Wheat Bran, 99% fat free, Trader Joe's | 1 | 110 | 0.5 | 0.0 | 0.0 | 23.0 | 8.0 |
| Blueberry, Dunkin' Donuts | 1 | 470 | 17.0 | 3.0 | 0.0 | 73.0 | 38.0 |
| ■ Reduced fat | 1 | 400 | 5.0 | 2.0 | 0.0 | 78.0 | 33.0 |
| Chocolate Chip, Dunkin' Donuts | 1 | 630 | 26.0 | 8.0 | 0.0 | 89.0 | 49.0 |
| Chocolate Chip, Little Bites, Entenmann's | 1 pouch | 210 | 10.0 | 2.0 | 0.0 | 28.0 | 18.0 |
| ■ Corn, Dunkin' Donuts | 1 | 510 | 18.0 | 3.5 | 0.0 | 77.0 | 32.0 |
| Cornbread, from mix, Jiffy | 1 muffin | 180 | 4.5 | 2.0 | 0.0 | 27.0 | 7.0 |
| Cranberry Orange, Dunkin' Donuts | 1 | 440 | 17.0 | 3.0 | 0.0 | 66.0 | 30.0 |
| ■ English Muffin, plain, Thomas' | 1 | 132 | 0.9 | 0.2 | 0.0 | 26.0 | n/a |
| ■ Cinnamon Raisin, Pepperidge Farm | 1 | 140 | 1.0 | 0.0 | 0.0 | 28.0 | 6.0 |
| ■ Whole wheat, Pepperidge Farm | 1 | 130 | 0.5 | 0.0 | 0.0 | 26.0 | 4.0 |
| * Pumpkin | 1 | 164 | 3.5 | 0.22 | 0.0 | n/a | n/a |
| ■ Sourdough | 1 | 130 | 1.0 | 0.0 | 0.0 | 26.0 | 1.0 |
| Honey Bran Raisin, Dunkin' Donuts | 1 | 480 | 15.0 | 2.5 | 0.0 | 79.0 | 43.0 |
| **Rolls** | | | | | | | |
| Cinnamon Rolls, Pillsbury, reduced fat | 1 | 140 | 3.5 | 1.0 | 1.5 | 24.0 | 10.0 |
| Crescent, Pillsbury | 1 | 110 | 6.0 | 1.5 | 1.5 | 11.0 | 2.0 |
| Reduced fat | 1 | 100 | 4.5 | 1.0 | 0.0 | 12.0 | 3.0 |
| Croissant, butter | 1 | 231 | 12.0 | 6.7 | 1.0 | 26.1 | 6.4 |

■ Contains less than 20% fat
n/a Not available

6

* See note, page xli

| Item | SERVING | CAL-ORIES | FAT GRAMS | SAT. FAT GRAMS | TRANS FAT GRAMS | CARB. GRAMS | SUGAR GRAMS |
|---|---|---|---|---|---|---|---|
| Cheese | 1 | 240 | 15.0 | 3.0 | n/a | 28.0 | 4.0 |
| Mini | 1 | 115 | 6.0 | 3.3 | 0.0 | 13.0 | 3.2 |
| Trader Joe's | 1 | 340 | 20.0 | 13.0 | 0.0 | 32.0 | 4.0 |
| ■ Dinner, small | 1 | 50 | 1.0 | 0.3 | 0.0 | 7.3 | 1.3 |
| Whole wheat, large | 1 | 96 | 1.7 | 0.3 | 0.0 | 18.4 | 3.1 |
| ■ French, Pepperidge Farm | 1 | 130 | 1.5 | 1.0 | 0.0 | 25.0 | 1.0 |
| ■ Hamburger bun | 1 | 120 | 1.9 | 0.5 | 0.0 | 21.3 | 2.7 |
| Whole wheat | 1 | 114 | 2.0 | 0.4 | 0.0 | 22.0 | 3.6 |
| ■ Hard rolls | 1 | 150 | 0.5 | 0.0 | 0.0 | 33.0 | 1.0 |
| ■ Hot dog bun | 1 | 120 | 1.9 | 0.5 | 0.0 | 21.3 | 2.7 |
| Reduced calorie | 1 | 84 | 0.9 | 0.1 | 0.0 | 18.1 | 2.7 |
| ■ Italian Brown & Serve | 1 | 130 | 2.0 | 1.0 | 0.0 | 24.0 | 1.0 |
| ■ Sourdough | 1 | 123 | 1.4 | 0.3 | 0.0 | 23.4 | 0.5 |
| **Stuffing** | | | | | | | |
| Chicken flavor, Stove Top | ½ cup | 170 | 18.0 | 3.0 | n/a | 42.0 | 6.0 |
| Cornbread | ½ cup | 300 | 19 | 9.0 | 0.0 | 28.0 | 3.0 |
| Seasoned | ¾ cup | 220 | 16.0 | 3.0 | n/a | 38.0 | 6.0 |
| Turkey flavor | ½ cup | 170 | 18.0 | 3.0 | n/a | 40.0 | 6.0 |
| **Other Breadstuffs** | | | | | | | |
| Boboli, thin crust | ⅕ crust | 170 | 3.5 | 1.5 | 0.0 | 28.0 | 1.0 |
| ■ Bread crumbs, plain | 1 oz. | 111 | 1.5 | 0.0 | 0.0 | 19.2 | 1.0 |
| ■ Italian style | 1 oz. | 111 | 1.5 | 0.0 | 0.0 | 20.3 | 1.0 |
| ■ Breadsticks, brown & serve | 1 each | 150 | 1.5 | 0.5 | 0.0 | 28.0 | 2.0 |
| ■ Corn flake crumbs | ¼ cup | 80 | 0.0 | 0.0 | 0.0 | 18.0 | 2.0 |
| ■ Crepe | 1 | 30 | 0.5 | 0.0 | 0.0 | 5.0 | 2.0 |
| ■ Croutons, plain | ¼ cup | 31 | 0.5 | 0.1 | 0.0 | 5.5 | n/a |
| Seasoned | 9 pieces | 33 | 1.3 | 0.3 | 0.0 | 4.3 | n/a |
| Filo dough shells, Athens | 2 | 45 | 2.0 | 0.0 | 0.0 | 5.0 | 0.0 |
| Hush puppies | 1 | 74 | 3.0 | 0.5 | 0.0 | 10.1 | 0.5 |
| Matzo ball mix, Manischewitz | 2 each | 50 | 0.0 | 0.0 | 0.0 | 11.0 | 0.0 |
| ■ Matzo meal | ¼ cup | 115 | 0.3 | 0.0 | 0.0 | 27.0 | 0.5 |
| ■ Panko, Honey, Orchid's | ⅓ cup | 70 | 0.5 | 0.0 | 0.0 | 15.0 | 2.0 |
| Pappadums | 1 | 50 | 3.0 | 0.0 | 0.0 | 5.0 | n/a |
| ■ Pizza crust | ⅛ crust | 94 | 1.3 | 0.0 | 0.0 | 16.9 | 1.9 |
| Puff pastry shells | 1 shell | 190 | 13.0 | 5.0 | 5.0 | 16.0 | 2.0 |
| Tortillas | | | | | | | |
| ■ Corn, 4.5" | 1 | 32 | 0.5 | 0.0 | 0.0 | 5.9 | 0.0 |
| ■ Corn, 6" | 1 | 70 | 1.0 | 0.0 | 0.0 | 14.0 | 0.0 |
| Flour, 6" | 1 | 90 | 3.0 | 0.0 | 0.0 | 13.0 | 0.0 |
| ■ Flour, 8" Tortilla Rica | 1 | 140 | 4.0 | 0.5 | 0.0 | 23.0 | 0.0 |
| ■ Low fat | 1 | 110 | 1.5 | 0.0 | 0.0 | 22.0 | 0.0 |
| ■ Whole wheat, 8" | 1 | 130 | 2 | 0.0 | 0.0 | 25.0 | 3.0 |
| Taco shells, white corn, Ortega | 2 | 120 | 6.0 | 1.0 | 0.0 | 16.0 | 0.0 |
| ■ Wonton wrappers | 1 | 23 | 0.1 | 0.0 | 0.0 | 4.6 | n/a |
| Zwieback | 1 piece | 30 | 0.7 | 0.3 | 0.0 | 5.2 | 1.2 |

■ Contains less than 20% fat
n/a Not available

| Item | SERVING | CALORIES | FAT GRAMS | SAT. FAT GRAMS | TRANS FAT GRAMS | CARB. GRAMS | SUGAR GRAMS |
|---|---|---|---|---|---|---|---|

## BREAKFAST FOODS
### Cereals

| Item | SERVING | CALORIES | FAT GRAMS | SAT. FAT GRAMS | TRANS FAT GRAMS | CARB. GRAMS | SUGAR GRAMS |
|---|---|---|---|---|---|---|---|
| ■ Amaranth Flakes, Arrowhead | 1 cup | 140 | 2.0 | 0.0 | 0.0 | 26.0 | 4.0 |
| ■ Basic 4 | 1 cup | 202 | 2.8 | 0.4 | 0.0 | 42.4 | 13.8 |
| Bran | | | | | | | |
| ■ 100% Bran | 1/3 cup | 83 | 0.6 | 0.1 | 0.0 | 22.7 | 7.1 |
| ■ All-Bran | 1/2 cup | 78 | 1.5 | 0.2 | 0.0 | 22.3 | 4.7 |
| ■ w/extra fiber | 1/2 cup | 58 | 1.1 | 0.2 | 0.0 | 23.1 | 0.1 |
| ■ Bran Flakes, Arrowhead | 1 cup | 110 | 1.0 | 0.0 | 0.0 | 22.0 | 3.0 |
| ■ Complete Wheat Bran Flakes | 1/2 cup | 61 | 0.4 | 0.1 | 0.0 | 15.3 | 3.3 |
| ■ Fiber One | 1/2 cup | 59 | 0.8 | 0.1 | 0.0 | 24.3 | 0.0 |
| ■ Oat bran, Quaker Oats, dry | 1/2 cup | 146 | 3.2 | 0.6 | 0.0 | 25.2 | 0.6 |
| ■ Raisin Bran, Kellogg's | 1 cup | 195 | 1.5 | 0.3 | 0.0 | 46.5 | 19.5 |
| ■ Skinner's | 1 cup | 170 | 1.0 | 0.0 | 0.0 | 41.0 | 13.0 |
| ■ Wheat, crude | 1 oz. | 61 | 1.2 | 0.2 | 0.0 | 18.3 | 0.1 |
| ■ Cheerios | 1 cup | 111 | 1.8 | 0.4 | 0.0 | 22.2 | 1.7 |
| ■ Honey Nut | 1 cup | 112 | 1.2 | 0.2 | 0.0 | 24.0 | 10.5 |
| ■ Multigrain | 1 cup | 108 | 1.2 | 0.3 | 0.0 | 24.3 | 6.0 |
| ■ Chex, Corn | 1.25 cup | 140 | 0.3 | 0.1 | 0.0 | 32.3 | 4.0 |
| ■ Corn Flakes | 1 cup | 101 | 0.2 | 0.1 | 0.0 | 24.4 | 2.9 |
| ■ Cornmeal, yellow, degermed, dry | 1/3 cup | 161 | 0.8 | 0.2 | 0.0 | 37.5 | 0.5 |
| ■ Corn Pops | 1 cup | 118 | 0.2 | 0.1 | 0.1 | 27.9 | 14.0 |
| ■ Crispix | 1 cup | 109 | 0.2 | 0.1 | 0.0 | 24.9 | 3.0 |
| ■ Crispy Brown Rice, Erewhon | 1 cup | 110 | 0.0 | 0.0 | 0.0 | 25.0 | 1.0 |
| ■ Farina, cooked | 1 cup | 125 | 0.5 | 0.1 | 0.0 | 26.9 | 0.2 |
| ■ Fiber 7, multigrain flakes | 3/4 cup | 100 | 0.0 | 0.0 | 0.0 | 24.0 | 5.0 |
| ■ Flax and Fiber Crunch, Back to Nature | 1 cup | 200 | 3.0 | 0.0 | 0.0 | 41.0 | 9.0 |
| ■ Flax Plus, organic, Nature's Path | 3/4 cup | 100 | 1.5 | 0.0 | 0.0 | 22.0 | 6.0 |
| ■ Froot Loops | 1 cup | 118 | 0.9 | 0.5 | 0.0 | 26.2 | 12.4 |
| ■ Frosted Flakes | 1 cup | 152 | 0.2 | 0.1 | 0.0 | 37.3 | 15.7 |
| ■ Fruit & Fibre, dates, raisins, & walnuts | 1 cup | 212 | 3.1 | 0.4 | 0.0 | 41.9 | 16.4 |
| ■ Go Lean, Kashi | 3/4 cup | 114 | 0.8 | 0.2 | 0.0 | 23.2 | 4.8 |
| ■ Golden Grahams | 3/4 cup | 112 | 1.1 | 0.2 | 0.0 | 24.9 | 10.5 |
| ■ Good Friends, Kashi | 3/4 cup | 95 | 1.1 | 0.1 | 0.0 | 24.5 | 5.1 |
| ■ Grainshop, Barbara's | 1/2 cup | 90 | 1.0 | 0.0 | 0.0 | 24.0 | 5.0 |
| Granola | | | | | | | |
| ■ Health Valley, date/almond, low fat | 2/3 cup | 190 | 2.0 | 0.0 | 0.0 | 42.0 | 10.0 |
| *■ Homemade | 1/2 cup | 208 | 2.2 | 0.5 | 0.0 | n/a | n/a |
| ■ Kellogg's, w/o raisins, low fat | 1/2 cup | 209 | 2.8 | 0.6 | 0.3 | 43.8 | 15.7 |
| ■ Quaker, 100% Natural, honey raisin oats | 1/2 cup | 225 | 8.6 | 3.6 | 0.0 | 34.4 | 16.1 |
| ■ Low fat | 2/3 cup | 213 | 3.0 | 0.8 | 0.0 | 44.3 | 18.3 |

■ Contains less than 20% fat
n/a Not available

8

* See note, page xli

| Item | SERVING | CAL-ORIES | FAT GRAMS | SAT. FAT GRAMS | TRANS FAT GRAMS | CARB. GRAMS | SUGAR GRAMS |
|---|---|---|---|---|---|---|---|
| ■ Grape Nuts | ⅓ cup | 137 | 0.7 | 0.2 | 0.0 | 31.1 | 4.6 |
| ■ Flakes | ⅓ cup | 47 | 0.4 | 0.1 | 0.0 | 10.4 | 2.3 |
| ■ Grits, corn, yellow, cooked | 1 cup | 143 | 0.5 | 0.1 | 0.0 | 31.2 | 0.2 |
| ■ Instant, plain, dry | 1 oz. | 97 | 0.3 | 0.0 | 0.0 | 22.3 | 0.1 |
| ■ Hi Protein Crunch, Back to Nature | ½ cup | 150 | 1.0 | 0.0 | 0.0 | 27.0 | 10.0 |
| ■ High Fiber, Trader Joe's | ⅔ cup | 89 | 1.0 | 0.0 | 0.0 | 24.8 | 5.9 |
| ■ Kamut Flakes, Arrowhead | 1 cup | 120 | 1.0 | 0.5 | 0.0 | 25.0 | 2.0 |
| ■ Kix | 1 cup | 85 | 0.5 | 0.1 | 0.0 | 19.4 | 2.5 |
| ■ Life, plain | 1 cup | 160 | 1.9 | 0.4 | 0.0 | 33.3 | 8.3 |
| ■ Cinnamon | 1 cup | 188 | 2.0 | 0.4 | 0.0 | 39.8 | 13.3 |
| ■ Mueslix, Swiss, Original | ½ cup | 220 | 3.0 | 0.5 | 0.0 | 41.0 | 14.0 |
| ■ No added sugar | ½ cup | 210 | 3.0 | 0.5 | 0.0 | 41.0 | 7.0 |
| ■ Oat Bran O's | ½ cup | 67 | 0.0 | 0.0 | 0.0 | 15.3 | 3.3 |
| ■ Oatmeal, plain, cooked | 1 cup | 147 | 2.3 | 0.4 | 0.0 | 25.3 | 3.4 |
| ■ Apple cinnamon, instant, Quaker | 1 packet | 128 | 1.5 | 0.3 | 0.0 | 27.3 | 12.4 |
| ■ Steel cut, dry, McCann's | ¼ cup | 150 | 2.0 | 0.0 | 0.0 | 26.0 | 0.0 |
| ■ Oatmeal Squares, Quaker | 1 cup | 212 | 2.4 | 0.5 | 0.0 | 43.9 | 9.0 |
| ■ Product 19 | 1 cup | 100 | 0.4 | 0.1 | 0.0 | 24.9 | 4.0 |
| ■ Puffed Millet, Arrowhead | 1 cup | 60 | 0.5 | 0.0 | 0.0 | 11.0 | 0.0 |
| ■ Puffed rice | 1 oz. | 109 | 0.3 | 0.1 | 0.0 | 24.9 | 0.0 |
| ■ Puffins, Barbara's | ¾ cup | 90 | 1.0 | 0.0 | 0.0 | 23.0 | 5.0 |
| ■ Rice Chex | 1.25 cup | 117 | 0.3 | 0.1 | 0.0 | 26.7 | 2.5 |
| ■ Rice Krispies | 1 cup | 95 | 0.3 | 0.1 | 0.0 | 22.4 | 2.9 |
| ■ Seven in the Morning, Kashi | ½ cup | 210 | 1.5 | 0.0 | 0.0 | 47.0 | 3.0 |
| ■ Smart Start | 1.25 cup | 228 | 0.9 | 0.2 | 0.0 | 53.8 | 17.5 |
| ■ Special K | 1 cup | 117 | 0.5 | 0.1 | 0.0 | 22.0 | 4.0 |
| ■ Total, wheat | 1 cup | 130 | 1.0 | 0.2 | 0.0 | 30.0 | 6.3 |
| ■ Trix | 1 cup | 117 | 1.1 | 0.2 | 0.0 | 26.7 | 13.2 |
| Uncle Sam's US Mills | 1 cup | 190 | 5.0 | 0.5 | 0.0 | 38.0 | <1.0 |
| Vanilla almond clusters, Trader Joe's | 1 cup | 220 | 6.0 | 0.5 | 0.0 | 38.0 | 11.0 |
| Weight Watcher's Flakes and Fiber w/Oats | ½ cup | 90 | 2.0 | 0.0 | 0.0 | 17.0 | 1.0 |
| Wheat | | | | | | | |
| ■ Arrowhead | 1 cup | 190 | 1.0 | 0.0 | 0.0 | 38.0 | 2.0 |
| ■ Biscuits, Quaker | 2 each | 144 | 0.8 | 0.3 | 0.0 | 33.6 | 0.3 |
| ■ Chex | ¾ cup | 78 | 0.5 | 0.1 | 0.0 | 18.2 | 2.3 |
| ■ Germ, Kretschmer | 2 tb. | 48 | 1.2 | 0.2 | 0.0 | 6.4 | n/a |
| ■ Puffed | 1 cup | 44 | 0.3 | 0.1 | 0.0 | 9.2 | 0.2 |
| ■ Wheat Hearts, dry | 1 oz. | 105 | 0.9 | 0.2 | 0.0 | 20.1 | 0.6 |
| ■ Wheatena, cooked | 1 cup | 136 | 1.2 | 0.2 | 0.0 | 28.7 | 0.6 |
| ■ Wheaties | 1 cup | 107 | 1.0 | 0.2 | 0.0 | 24.3 | 4.2 |
| ■ Wheat 'N Bran, Original, Post | 1.25 cup | 197 | 0.8 | 0.1 | 0.0 | 47.1 | 0.6 |

■ Contains less than 20% fat
n/a Not available

| Item | SERVING | CAL-ORIES | FAT GRAMS | SAT. FAT GRAMS | TRANS FAT GRAMS | CARB. GRAMS | SUGAR GRAMS |
|---|---|---|---|---|---|---|---|
| **Pancakes** | | | | | | | |
| Aunt Jemima, Buttermilk mix | 1/3 cup | 160 | 2.0 | 0.0 | 0.0 | 31.0 | 6.0 |
| Bisquick, dry | 1/3 cup | 163 | 6.1 | 1.6 | 1.5 | 24.7 | 0.7 |
| ■ Reduced fat | 1/3 cup | 152 | 2.5 | 0.5 | 0.5 | 28.3 | 2.0 |
| ■ Krusteaz, original, frozen | 3 each | 280 | 4.0 | 5.0 | 0.0 | 52.0 | 11.0 |
| ■ Blueberry, frozen | 2 each | 166 | 2.7 | n/a | n/a | 30.9 | n/a |
| ■ Krusteaz, buckwheat mix | 2 each | 227 | 3.3 | 0.7 | 0.0 | 42.0 | 5.3 |
| Pancake Syrup | | | | | | | |
| ■ Hungry Jack, light | 1/4 cup | 100 | 0.0 | 0.0 | 0.0 | 24.0 | 23.0 |
| ■ Log Cabin | 1/4 cup | 200 | 0.0 | 0.0 | 0.0 | 52.0 | 31.0 |
| ■ Light, reduced calorie | 1/4 cup | 100 | 0.0 | 0.0 | 0.0 | 26.0 | 25.0 |
| ■ Maple | 1/4 cup | 209 | 0.2 | 0.0 | 0.0 | 53.7 | 47.6 |
| **Waffles** | | | | | | | |
| ■ Belgian, frozen, Private Selection | 1 piece | 200 | 9.0 | 1.0 | 0.0 | 26.0 | 7.0 |
| Waffles | | | | | | | |
| ■ Aunt Jemima, whole grain, frozen | 1 each | 77 | 1.4 | 0.4 | 0.0 | 14.7 | n/a |
| Eggo, Nutrí Grain, frozen | 2 each | 180 | 6.0 | 1.0 | 1.0 | 22.0 | 3.0 |
| Eggo, homestyle, frozen | 2 each | 190 | 6.0 | 1.5 | 2.0 | 29.0 | 2.0 |
| Hungry Jack, homestyle, frozen | 1 each | 90 | 3.0 | 1.0 | n/a | 14.5 | 2.0 |
| Lifestream Flax Plus | 2 pieces | 240 | 9.0 | 1.0 | 0.0 | 34.0 | 5.0 |
| ■ Oat bran, homemade | 1/2 piece | 174 | 4.1 | <1* | 0.0 | n/a | n/a |
| ■ Special K, fat free, frozen | 2 each | 120 | 0.0 | 0.0 | 0.0 | 26.0 | 3.0 |
| **Other Breakfast Foods** **(see also Breads, Sweetened; Eggs, Egg Dishes, & Egg Substitutes)** | | | | | | | |
| Blintz, Cheese, Old Fashioned Kitchen | 1 | 100 | 1.5 | 0.5 | 0.0 | 14.0 | 4.0 |
| Breakfast Bars | | | | | | | |
| Carnation, chocolate chip, chewy | 1 | 150 | 6.0 | 2.0 | 0.0 | 24.0 | 11.0 |
| ■ Entenmann's, strawberry | 1 | 140 | 3.0 | 1.5 | 0.0 | 26.0 | 15.0 |
| ■ Health Valley, blueberry cobbler | 1 | 130 | 2.0 | 0.0 | 0.0 | 27.0 | 13.0 |
| ■ Strawberry filled, low fat | 1 | 134 | 2.1 | 0.0 | 0.0 | 27.7 | 13.4 |
| ■ Kashi, Go Lean | 1 | 170 | 4.0 | 1.5 | 0.0 | 30.0 | 13.0 |
| Nutri Grain, apple cinnamon | 1 | 136 | 2.8 | 0.6 | 0.0 | 27.0 | n/a |
| Breakfast Treat, Stella D'oro | 1 | 90 | 3.0 | 0.5 | n/a | 15.0 | 6.0 |
| *■ Burrito, Breakfast | 1 | 187 | 3.8 | 3.3 | 0.0 | n/a | n/a |
| w/sausage, Great Starts, Swanson | 1 each | 240 | 12.0 | 4.0 | n/a | 24.0 | 2.0 |
| Eggs, scrambled w/bacon, Great Starts, Swanson | 1 each | 290 | 19.0 | 9.0 | n/a | 17.0 | 2.0 |
| English Muffin Sandwich, Smart Ones | 1 | 210 | 5.0 | 3.0 | 0.0 | 28.0 | 1.0 |

■ Contains less than 20% fat
n/a Not available

* See note, page xli

| Item | SERVING | CAL-ORIES | FAT GRAMS | SAT. FAT GRAMS | TRANS FAT GRAMS | CARB. GRAMS | SUGAR GRAMS |
|---|---|---|---|---|---|---|---|
| * French Toast, frozen | 2 pieces | 166 | 4.4 | n/a | 0.0 | 26.5 | n/a |
| ■ Instant Breakfast, Carnation, milk chocolate | 1 can | 220 | 2.5 | 1.0 | 0.0 | 37.0 | 34.0 |
| ■ French vanilla | 1 can | 200 | 3.0 | 0.5 | 0.0 | 31.0 | 29.0 |
| ■ Strawberry crème | 1 can | 220 | 3.0 | 0.5 | 0.0 | 35.0 | 33.0 |
| Pop-Tart, Kellogg's apple cinnamon | 1 each | 205 | 5.3 | 0.9 | 0.0 | 37.5 | 17.5 |
| ■ Brown sugar cinnamon, low fat | 1 each | 188 | 2.8 | 0.6 | 0.0 | 39.2 | 18.1 |
| Sausage, pork, patty, cooked | 1 each | 92 | 7.7 | 2.5 | 0.1 | 0.0 | 0.0 |
| Vegetarian substitute, patty, Morningstar Farms | 1 each | 79 | 2.8 | 0.5 | 0.0 | 3.7 | 0.6 |
| Scone, currant, Trader Joe's | 1 | 330 | 18.0 | 11.0 | 0.5 | 36.0 | 9.0 |
| ■ Toaster Pastry, Nature's Path, strawberry, frosted | 1 | 210 | 4.0 | 2.0 | 0.0 | 40.0 | 19.0 |
| ■ unfrosted | 1 | 210 | 4.5 | 2.0 | 0.0 | 40.0 | 18.0 |
| Toaster Strudel, apple spice, Pillsbury, frozen | 1 each | 200 | 9.0 | 1.5 | 1.0 | 26.0 | 10.0 |

## CANDY

| Item | SERVING | CAL-ORIES | FAT GRAMS | SAT. FAT GRAMS | TRANS FAT GRAMS | CARB. GRAMS | SUGAR GRAMS |
|---|---|---|---|---|---|---|---|
| Almond Bar | | | | | | | |
| Dark chocolate, Toblerone | 1 oz. | 153 | 10.0 | 5.3 | 0.0 | 15.3 | 12.7 |
| Golden Almond, Hershey's | 3.5 oz. bar | 480 | 30.5 | 18.0 | 0.0 | 60.0 | 45.0 |
| Almond Joy | 1.7 oz. bar | 231 | 13.0 | 8.5 | 0.0 | 28.7 | 23.3 |
| Almonds, chocolate-coated | 1 oz. | 156 | 12.1 | 4.3 | 0.0 | 12.8 | 8.5 |
| Sugar-coated | 1 oz. | 134 | 5.0 | 0.5 | n/a | 19.5 | 17.7 |
| Baby Ruth | 2.1 oz. bar | 276 | 14.9 | 7.3 | 0.0 | 36.8 | 27.6 |
| Bridge mix, Brach's | 16 pieces | 190 | 8.0 | 4.5 | n/a | 26.0 | 22.0 |
| Butterfinger | 2.16 oz. bar | 291 | 11.6 | 6.3 | n/a | 44.4 | 32.1 |
| ■ Butterscotch | 1 oz. | 111 | 0.9 | 0.6 | 0.0 | 25.6 | 25.6 |
| ■ Candied Fruit, Citron | 1 oz. | 85 | 0.0 | 0.0 | 0.0 | 21.7 | 16.1 |
| ■ Candy corn | 1 oz. | 106 | 0.0 | 0.0 | 0.0 | 26.5 | 26.5 |
| ■ Candy, hard | 1 oz. | 112 | 0.1 | 0.0 | 0.0 | 27.8 | 17.8 |
| ■ Caramel | 1 piece | 39 | 0.8 | 0.7 | 0.0 | 7.8 | 6.6 |
| Caramel roll, chocolate-coated, Rolo | 3 pieces | 43 | 1.9 | 1.3 | 0.0 | 6.1 | 5.8 |
| Chocolate, cooking | | | | | | | |
| Bittersweet | 1 oz. | 142 | 12.2 | 6.1 | 0.0 | 14.2 | 10.1 |
| Semisweet | 1 oz. | 122 | 7.1 | 4.1 | 0.0 | 18.2 | 16.2 |
| Sweet | 1 oz. | 131 | 7.6 | 4.4 | 0.0 | 17.5 | 15.5 |
| Chocolate bar | | | | | | | |
| Dark, Dove | 1.3 oz. bar | 200 | 12.0 | 7.0 | 0.0 | 22.0 | 19.0 |
| Newman's Own | ½ bar | 200 | 13.0 | 7.0 | 0.0 | 24.0 | 20.0 |
| Plain, milk, Hershey's | 1 each | 90 | 5.0 | 3.5 | 0.0 | 10.0 | 8.7 |
| Miniatures | 1 each | 45 | 2.5 | 1.5 | 0.0 | 5.0 | 4.4 |
| w/almonds, Hershey's | 1 each | 100 | 6.0 | 3.0 | 0.0 | 9.0 | 7.1 |
| Cadbury | 9 pieces | 198 | 11.7 | 6.3 | 0.0 | 18.9 | 16.2 |

■ Contains less than 20% fat
n/a Not available

11

* See note, page xli

| Item | SERVING | CAL-ORIES | FAT GRAMS | SAT. FAT GRAMS | TRANS FAT GRAMS | CARB. GRAMS | SUGAR GRAMS |
|---|---|---|---|---|---|---|---|
| Scharffen Berger | 0.5 bar | 260 | 19.0 | 12.0 | n/a | 18.0 | 9.0 |
| Special Dark, Hershey's | 4 pieces | 115 | 7.0 | 4.2 | 0.0 | 12.8 | 10.3 |
| Dove Promises | 5 pieces | 210 | 13.0 | 8.0 | 0.0 | 24.0 | 20.0 |
| Fudge | | | | | | | |
| Chocolate | 1 oz. | 124 | 5.3 | 3.3 | 0.0 | 18.7 | 18.0 |
| w/nuts | 1 oz. | 131 | 5.4 | 1.7 | 0.0 | 19.3 | 18.1 |
| ■ Vanilla | 1 oz. | 109 | 1.5 | 0.8 | 0.0 | 23.3 | 23.3 |
| w/nuts | 1 oz. | 123 | 3.9 | 0.9 | 0.0 | 21.2 | 20.8 |
| ■ Good & Plenty | 1 oz. | 100 | 0.0 | 0.0 | 0.0 | 23.4 | 15.0 |
| Gum | | | | | | | |
| ■ Care Free | 1 piece | 5 | 0.0 | 0.0 | 0.0 | 2.0 | 0.0 |
| ■ Dentyne Ice | 1 piece | 3 | 0.0 | 0.0 | 0.0 | 2.0 | 0.0 |
| ■ Doublemint, Wrigley | 1 piece | 10 | 0.0 | 0.0 | 0.0 | 2.0 | 2.0 |
| ■ Trident | 1 piece | 5 | 0.0 | 0.0 | 0.0 | 1.0 | 0.0 |
| ■ Gumdrops | 1 oz. | 112 | 0.0 | 0.0 | 0.0 | 28.0 | 16.7 |
| Halvah | 1 oz. | 131 | 6.0 | 1.1 | n/a | 16.9 | 15.7 |
| Heath Bar | 1 bar | 110 | 12.0 | 5.0 | n/a | 24.0 | 23.0 |
| ■ Jellybeans, small | 1 oz. | 106 | 0.0 | 0.0 | 0.0 | 26.5 | 19.8 |
| Kisses, Hershey's | 1 oz. | 145 | 8.7 | 5.2 | 0.0 | 16.8 | n/a |
| Kit Kat | 1.5 oz. bar | 220 | 11.1 | 7.6 | 0.0 | 27.5 | 20.7 |
| Kudos, peanut butter | 1 each | 130 | 5.0 | 2.0 | n/a | 19.0 | 13.0 |
| ■ Licorice, Twizzlers | 1 oz. | 30 | 0.0 | 0.0 | 0.0 | 7.0 | 4.0 |
| ■ Lifesavers, regular | 1 piece | 9 | 0.0 | 0.0 | 0.0 | 2.3 | n/a |
| M&M's | | | | | | | |
| Peanut | 1.67 oz. bag | 146 | 7.4 | 2.9 | 0.0 | 17.1 | 14.4 |
| Fun size | 1 each | 108 | 5.5 | 2.2 | 0.0 | 12.7 | 10.7 |
| Plain chocolate | 1.48 oz. box | 139 | 6.0 | 3.7 | 0.0 | 20.2 | 18.1 |
| Malt Balls, Milk Chocolate | 1 oz. | 135 | 7.1 | 4.3 | 0.0 | 18.4 | 9.9 |
| Mars Bar | 1.76 oz. bar | 234 | 11.5 | 3.6 | n/a | 31.4 | 26.1 |
| ■ Marshmallows | 1 oz. | 90 | 0.1 | 0.0 | 0.0 | 23.1 | 16.3 |
| Milky Way | 2.1 oz. bar | 252 | 9.6 | 4.6 | 0.0 | 42.7 | 36.1 |
| Milky Way Lite | 1.57 oz. bar | 170 | 5.0 | n/a | 0.0 | 30.0 | n/a |
| Mints | | | | | | | |
| Chocolate covered, After Eight | 5 pieces | 147 | 5.6 | 3.4 | 0.0 | 31.5 | n/a |
| ■ York Peppermint Pattie | 1 | 160 | 3.0 | 1.4 | n/a | 32.0 | 25.0 |
| Mounds | 1.9 oz. bar | 262 | 14.3 | 11.1 | 0.0 | 31.6 | 24.9 |
| Mr. Goodbar | 1.75 oz. bar | 267 | 16.5 | 7.0 | n/a | 27.0 | 23.4 |
| Nestlé Crunch | 1.4 oz. bar | 207 | 10.4 | 6.0 | 0.0 | 25.9 | 22.2 |
| Peanuts, chocolate-coated | 1 oz. | 147 | 9.5 | 4.1 | n/a | 14.0 | 10.7 |
| Oh Henry! | 2 oz. bar | 262 | 13.1 | 3.8 | n/a | 37.1 | 28.4 |
| Reese's Peanut Butter Cups | 1 each | 88 | 5.2 | 1.8 | 0.0 | 9.4 | 8.0 |
| ■ Popcorn, Cracker Jacks, original | ½ cup | 120 | 2.0 | 0.0 | 0.0 | 23.0 | 15.0 |
| ■ Caramel, fat free | ½ cup | 73 | 0.0 | 0.0 | 0.0 | 17.3 | 11.3 |
| Raisins, carob coated | 1 oz. | 120 | 3.5 | 3.5 | 0.0 | 21.3 | 13.5 |
| Raisins, milk chocolate coated | 1 oz. | 111 | 4.2 | 2.5 | 0.0 | 19.4 | 17.6 |

■ Contains less than 20% fat
n/a Not available

| Item | SERVING | CAL-ORIES | FAT GRAMS | SAT. FAT GRAMS | TRANS FAT GRAMS | CARB. GRAMS | SUGAR GRAMS |
|---|---|---|---|---|---|---|---|
| Snickers | 2 oz. bar | 265 | 10.9 | 4.2 | 0.2 | 36.6 | 28.3 |
| Fun size | 1 each | 70 | 2.9 | 1.1 | 0.0 | 9.7 | 7.5 |
| 3 Musketeers | 1.8 oz. bar | 214 | 6.6 | 3.3 | 0.0 | 39.5 | 34.0 |
| ■ Tootsie Roll | 1 oz. | 110 | 0.9 | 0.3 | 0.0 | 24.9 | 16.0 |
| Turtles, chocolate caramel pecans | 2 pieces | 165 | 9.5 | 3.7 | 0.0 | 19.7 | 13.3 |
| Twix, caramel | 2 oz. bar | 283 | 13.8 | 5.1 | 0.0 | 37.2 | 27.2 |

## COOKIES

| Item | SERVING | CAL-ORIES | FAT GRAMS | SAT. FAT GRAMS | TRANS FAT GRAMS | CARB. GRAMS | SUGAR GRAMS |
|---|---|---|---|---|---|---|---|
| ■ Almond Toast, Stella D'Oro | 3 | 115 | 2.5 | 0.5 | 0.0 | 21.0 | 10.0 |
| Animal crackers, Barnum's | 10 | 130 | 3.5 | 1.0 | 0.0 | 22.0 | 7.0 |
| Arrowroot, adult, Nabisco | 1 | 20 | 0.5 | 0.2 | 0.0 | 3.0 | n/a |
| Biscotti, plain, Perugina | 1 | 120 | 5.0 | 2.0 | n/a | 17.0 | 9.0 |
| Chocolate dipped, Pepperidge Farm | 1 | 110 | 4.0 | 2.0 | n/a | 14.0 | 6.0 |
| Bordeaux, Pepperidge Farm | 1 | 33 | 1.3 | 0.6 | 0.0 | 5.0 | 3.0 |
| Brownie, 2" homemade | 1 | 243 | 10.1 | 3.1 | 0.0 | 39.0 | n/a |
| w/nuts | 1 | 340 | 13.0 | n/a | 0.0 | 55.0 | n/a |
| Little Debbie, fudge | 1 | 270 | 12.0 | 3.0 | 3.5 | 39.0 | 22.0 |
| Entenmann's Little Bites, fudge, mini | 3 | 300 | 16.0 | 2.5 | 0.0 | 36.0 | 25.0 |
| Café Twists, Trader Joe's | 1 | 60 | 2.0 | 0.5 | 0.0 | 9.0 | 4.0 |
| Cameo, sandwich cream, Nabisco | 1 | 65 | 2.5 | 0.5 | 0.8 | 10.5 | 5.0 |
| Chessman, Pepperidge Farm | 1 | 40 | 1.7 | 1.0 | 0.0 | 6.0 | 1.7 |
| Chocolate chip, Keebler | 1 | 80 | 4.0 | 1.0 | 1.5 | 9.0 | 4.0 |
| ■ Health Valley, double chocolate, fat free | 3 | 100 | 0.0 | 0.0 | 0.0 | 24.0 | 11.0 |
| Homemade | 1 | 78 | 4.5 | 2.3 | n/a | 9.3 | n/a |
| Pepperidge Farm, Old Fashioned | 1 | 53 | 2.3 | 0.8 | 0.0 | 6.0 | 3.0 |
| Refrigerated cookie dough, Pillsbury | 1 | 127 | 5.7 | 1.8 | n/a | 17.9 | 10.4 |
| w/walnuts | 1 | 163 | 8.2 | 2.3 | n/a | 19.8 | 11.6 |
| Nestle's Toll House, Break & Bake | 1 | 110 | 5.0 | 2.0 | n/a | 16.0 | 10.0 |
| Snackwell's, low fat | 1 | 61 | 1.8 | 0.8 | n/a | 10.7 | 4.7 |
| Chocolate Creme, Keebler | 1 | 48 | 2.1 | 0.5 | n/a | 7.3 | 4.2 |
| Chocolate wafer, Nabisco | 1 | 28 | 0.8 | 0.3 | n/a | 4.8 | 2.2 |
| ■ Devil's food, Snackwell's, fat free | 1 | 49 | 0.2 | 0.1 | 0.0 | 11.9 | 6.9 |
| ■ Fig Newman's, Newman's Own, low fat | 2 | 140 | 2.0 | 1.0 | 0.0 | 28.0 | 13.0 |
| Fig Newton | 2 | 120 | 3.0 | 1.0 | 0.0 | 20.0 | 14.0 |
| ■ Apple | 2 | 144 | 0.0 | 0.0 | 0.0 | 32.0 | n/a |
| ■ Fat free | 2 | 136 | 0.0 | 0.0 | 0.0 | 31.2 | n/a |
| Gingersnap, Mi-Del | 5 | 130 | 4.0 | 0.0 | 0.0 | 22.0 | 11.0 |
| Girl Scout | | | | | | | |
| All Abouts | 2 | 130 | 6.0 | 3.0 | 0.0 | 17.0 | 8.0 |
| Café | 5 | 150 | 6.0 | 2.0 | 0.0 | 20.0 | 11.0 |

■ Contains less than 20% fat
n/a Not available

| Item | SERVING | CAL-ORIES | FAT GRAMS | SAT. FAT GRAMS | TRANS FAT GRAMS | CARB. GRAMS | SUGAR GRAMS |
|---|---|---|---|---|---|---|---|
| Do-Si-Dos | 2 | 110 | 5.0 | 1.5 | 0.0 | 15.0 | 8.0 |
| Little Brownie | 3 | 130 | 7.0 | 3.0 | 0.0 | 16.0 | 0.0 |
| Samoas | 2 | 150 | 8.0 | 4.0 | 0.0 | 19.0 | 11.0 |
| Tagalongs | 2 | 130 | 9.0 | 4.5 | 0.0 | 13.0 | 7.0 |
| Thin Mints | 4 | 160 | 8.0 | 6.0 | 0.0 | 22.0 | 11.0 |
| Graham crackers, amaranth, Health Valley | 4 | 80 | 2.0 | 0.0 | 0.0 | 14.7 | 2.7 |
| ■ Crispy, Keeber, low fat | 4 | 114 | 1.7 | 0.4 | 0.0 | 22.7 | 7.0 |
| Honey, Keebler | 4 | 122 | 3.4 | 0.9 | n/a | 21.0 | 6.2 |
| Lemon Snaps, Mi-Del | 5 | 140 | 4.5 | 0.0 | 0.0 | 21.0 | 10.0 |
| Lido, Pepperidge Farm | 1 | 90 | 4.5 | 1.5 | 0.0 | 11.0 | 5.0 |
| Macaroons, Archway | 1 | 106 | 6.1 | 5.4 | 0.0 | 12.4 | 9.5 |
| Milano, Pepperidge Farm | 3 | 180 | 10.0 | 3.5 | 0.0 | 21.0 | 11.0 |
| Molasses, big, Grandma's | 1 | 160 | 4.0 | 1.5 | 0.0 | 29.0 | 18.0 |
| Newman-O's Crème Filled Chocolate | 2 | 130 | 4.5 | 1.5 | 0.0 | 20.0 | 10.0 |
| Nilla Wafers | 8 | 140 | 5.0 | 1.0 | 0.0 | 24.0 | 12.0 |
| Nutty Bars, Little Debbie | 1 | 312 | 18.7 | 3.6 | 5.0 | 31.5 | 19.4 |
| Oatmeal, homemade | 1 | 67 | 2.7 | 0.5 | n/a | 10.0 | n/a |
| Oatmeal raisin, Archway | 1 | 43 | 2.0 | 0.5 | 0.5 | 6.3 | 3.3 |
| Grandma's big, homestyle | 1 | 160 | 6.0 | 1.5 | n/a | 26.0 | 15.0 |
| ■ Health Valley, fat free | 2 | 67 | 0.0 | 0.0 | 0.0 | 16.0 | 7.3 |
| Snackwell's, sugar free | 1 | 95 | 2.5 | 0.5 | n/a | 17.0 | 0.0 |
| Oreo | 2 | 107 | 4.7 | 1.0 | 1.7 | 15.3 | 8.7 |
| Double Stuff | 2 | 140 | 7.0 | 1.5 | 0.0 | 19.0 | 12.0 |
| Reduced fat | 2 | 96 | 2.4 | 0.6 | 0.0 | 17.4 | 9.4 |
| Peanut butter, homemade | 1 | 72 | 3.5 | 0.7 | 0.0 | 8.8 | 4.8 |
| Raspberry Chantilly, Pepperidge Farm | 2 | 160 | 6.0 | 1.0 | 0.0 | 24.0 | 14.0 |
| ■ Rice Krispies square | 1 | 91 | 2.0 | 0.3 | 0.0 | 17.7 | n/a |
| Shortbread, Lorna Doone | 4 | 140 | 7.0 | 1.5 | 0.0 | 19.0 | 6.0 |

## CRACKERS

| Item | SERVING | CAL-ORIES | FAT GRAMS | SAT. FAT GRAMS | TRANS FAT GRAMS | CARB. GRAMS | SUGAR GRAMS |
|---|---|---|---|---|---|---|---|
| ■ Ak-Mak | 5 | 122 | 0.3 | 0.1 | 0.0 | 25.6 | 0.8 |
| Better Cheddars, low sodium | 22 | 144 | 7.2 | 2.7 | n/a | 16.7 | 0.6 |
| Breton fat-reduced | 4 | 78 | 2.1 | 0.8 | 0.0 | 13.0 | 1.4 |
| ■ Brown Rice, Eden, Wheat Free | 8 | 120 | 2.0 | 0.0 | 0.0 | 22.0 | <1 |
| Carr's water | 5 | 70 | 1.5 | 0.5 | 0.0 | 13.0 | 0.0 |
| Cheese Bites, Barbara's Bakery | 22 | 120 | 3.0 | 0.5 | 0.0 | 20.0 | 1.0 |
| Cheese & Peanut Butter, Keebler | 1 | 181 | 8.7 | 1.7 | 1.0 | 21.7 | 3.8 |
| Cheese-It | 27 | 156 | 8.4 | 1.7 | 0.0 | 16.2 | 0.6 |
| ■ Finn, crispbread, rye | 3 | 22 | 0.1 | 0.0 | 0.0 | 4.9 | 0.4 |
| Goldfish, tiny, Pepperidge Farm | | | | | | | |
| Cheese, original cheese | 55 | 140 | 6.0 | 2.0 | 0.0 | 19.0 | 0.0 |
| Low sodium | 55 | 150 | 6.0 | 1.5 | 0.0 | 18.0 | 0.0 |
| Parmesan | 55 | 140 | 5.0 | n/a | 0.0 | 19.0 | 0.0 |
| Pizza | 55 | 140 | 6.0 | n/a | 0.0 | 19.0 | 1.0 |

■ Contains less than 20% fat
n/a Not available

| Item | SERVING | CAL-ORIES | FAT GRAMS | SAT. FAT GRAMS | TRANS FAT GRAMS | CARB. GRAMS | SUGAR GRAMS |
|---|---|---|---|---|---|---|---|
| ■ Pretzel | 55 | 120 | 2.5 | 1.0 | 0.0 | 22.0 | 1.0 |
| Hi Ho | 4 | 72 | 3.9 | 0.8 | n/a | 8.3 | 0.8 |
| Just Crisps, Just Off Melrose | 1-2 | 70 | 4.0 | 3.0 | n/a | 7.0 | 0.0 |
| ■ Kavli, crispy thin | 3 | 60 | 0.0 | 0.0 | 0.0 | 13.0 | 0.0 |
| Lavasch, Nejaimes | 0.5 | 70 | 2.0 | 0.0 | 0.0 | 10.0 | 1.0 |
| ■ Matzo, plain, board | 1 | 112 | 0.4 | 0.1 | 0.0 | 23.7 | 0.1 |
| Manischewitz | | | | | | | |
| ■ Egg | 1 | 120 | 1.0 | 0.5 | 0.0 | 25.0 | 1.0 |
| ■ Everything | 1 | 110 | 0.5 | 0.0 | 0.0 | 22.0 | 0.0 |
| ■ Thins | 1 | 100 | 0.0 | 0.0 | 0.0 | 22.0 | 1.0 |
| ■ Whole wheat | 1 | 100 | 0.4 | 0.1 | 0.0 | 22.4 | n/a |
| Manischewitz, crackers | | | | | | | |
| ■ Everything | 12 | 110 | 0.5 | 0.0 | 0.0 | 22.0 | 0.0 |
| Miniatures | 13 | 130 | 4.0 | 2.0 | n/a | 22.0 | 2.0 |
| Tams | 10 | 130 | 4.0 | 2.0 | n/a | 22.0 | 2.0 |
| ■ Melba toast, plain | 1 oz. | 111 | 0.9 | 0.1 | 0.0 | 21.7 | 0.3 |
| ■ pumpernickel | 5 | 97 | 0.9 | 0.1 | 0.0 | 19.3 | n/a |
| Oyster, small, Keebler | 1 package | 64 | 2.5 | 0.6 | 0.0 | 9.1 | 0.6 |
| Rice bran, Health Valley | 6 | 110 | 3.0 | 0.0 | 0.0 | 19.0 | 4.0 |
| ■ Rice cake, plain, Quaker | 1 | 35 | 0.3 | 0.1 | 0.0 | 7.5 | 0.1 |
| ■ Apple cinnamon, mini | 8 | 87 | 0.6 | 0.1 | 0.0 | 19.3 | 5.8 |
| ■ Lundberg Organic Brown Rice, salt-free | 1 | 70 | 0.0 | 0.0 | 0.0 | 16.0 | 0.0 |
| Ritz, Nabisco | 5 | 79 | 3.7 | 0.6 | 0.0 | 10.3 | 1.3 |
| Reduced fat | 5 | 70 | 2.0 | 0.0 | 0.0 | 11.0 | 1.0 |
| Ritz Bits, Nabisco | 14 | 47 | 2.6 | 0.3 | 0.0 | 5.3 | 1.2 |
| ■ Rye, wafer | 1 oz. | 104 | 0.4 | 0.0 | 0.0 | 23.3 | 0.3 |
| ■ Ry Krisp, Original | 2 | 60 | 0.0 | 0.0 | 0.0 | 13.0 | 0.0 |
| Seasoned | 2 | 60 | 1.5 | 0.0 | 0.0 | 10.0 | 0.0 |
| ■ Wasa crispbread | 1 | 31 | 0.1 | 0.0 | 0.0 | 7.0 | 0.5 |
| Saltines, Premium, Nabisco | 5 | 66 | 2.0 | 0.0 | 1.0 | 11.0 | 0.0 |
| ■ Fat free | 5 | 50 | 0.0 | 0.0 | 0.0 | 11.0 | 0.0 |
| ■ Low sodium | 5 | 73 | 1.9 | 0.0 | 0.0 | 12.5 | 0.0 |
| ■ Unsalted tops | 5 | 63 | 1.3 | n/a | 0.0 | 10.0 | 0.0 |
| ■ Wheatines, Barbara's Bakery | 4 | 60 | 1.0 | 0.0 | 0.0 | 11.0 | 1.0 |
| Sesame, Pepperidge Farms | 3 | 70 | 2.5 | 0.0 | 0.0 | 9.0 | 0.0 |
| Sociables | 7 | 98 | 4.9 | 0.7 | 0.0 | 12.6 | 1.4 |
| Soda | 1 oz. | 121 | 3.2 | 0.5 | 1.0 | 20.1 | 0.1 |
| Stoned Wheat Thins, Red Oval Farms | 2 | 60 | 1.5 | 0.0 | 0.0 | 11.0 | 0.0 |
| TLC, Original 7 Grain, Kashi | 15 | 130 | 3.0 | 0.0 | 0.0 | 22.0 | 3.0 |
| Triscuit | 7 | 150 | 6.0 | 1.0 | 0.0 | 21.0 | n/a |
| Low sodium | 6 | 130 | 5.0 | 1.0 | 0.0 | 19.0 | 0.0 |
| Reduced fat | 6 | 120 | 3.0 | 0.0 | 0.0 | 21.0 | 0.0 |
| Uneeda Biscuit, unsalted tops | 2 | 60 | 1.5 | 0.0 | 0.0 | 11.0 | 0.0 |
| ■ Water, Table, plain, and w/pepper, Carr's | 4 | 60 | 1.0 | 0.0 | 0.5 | 12.0 | 0.0 |

■ Contains less than 20% fat
n/a Not available

| Item | SERVING | CAL-ORIES | FAT GRAMS | SAT. FAT GRAMS | TRANS FAT GRAMS | CARB. GRAMS | SUGAR GRAMS |
|---|---|---|---|---|---|---|---|
| Wheat, Hearty, Pepperidge Farm | 3 | 80 | 3.5 | 0.0 | 0.0 | 10.0 | 2.0 |
| Wheatsworth | 5 | 80 | 3.5 | 0.5 | n/a | 10.0 | 0.0 |
| Wheat Thins, original | 16 | 136 | 5.8 | 0.9 | 0.0 | 20.0 | 2.6 |
| Low sodium | 16 | 147 | 5.9 | 2.0 | 0.0 | 21.7 | 0.5 |
| Reduced fat | 16 | 130 | 4.0 | 0.5 | 0.0 | 21.0 | 3.0 |
| ■ Whole grain, brown rice | 7 | 60 | 0.0 | 0.0 | 0.0 | 13.0 | 0.0 |
| Whole wheat, vegetable, Health Valley, unsalted, low fat | 5 | 50 | 1.3 | 0.0 | 0.0 | 8.3 | 0.8 |
| Zwieback | 1 oz. | 121 | 2.8 | 1.1 | 0.0 | 21.0 | 4.7 |

## DAIRY AND DAIRY PRODUCTS

### Cheese

**American**

| Item | SERVING | CAL-ORIES | FAT GRAMS | SAT. FAT GRAMS | TRANS FAT GRAMS | CARB. GRAMS | SUGAR GRAMS |
|---|---|---|---|---|---|---|---|
| Alpine Lace, 33% less fat, 50% less salt | 1 oz. | 80 | 6.0 | 4.0 | 0.0 | 2.0 | 0.0 |
| Kraft, reduced fat | 1 slice | 45 | 3.0 | 1.5 | 0.0 | 1.0 | 1.0 |
| ■ Kraft Free | 1 slice | 31 | 0.2 | 0.2 | 0.0 | 2.5 | 1.4 |
| ■ Smart Beat, lactose & fat free | 1 slice | 25 | 0.0 | 0.0 | 0.0 | 3.0 | 2.0 |
| Babybel, mini, original | 1 oz. | 70 | 6.0 | 4.0 | 0.0 | 0.0 | 0.0 |
| Light | 1 oz. | 50 | 3.0 | 1.5 | 0.0 | 0.0 | 0.0 |
| Blue | 1 oz. | 100 | 8.2 | 5.3 | 0.0 | 0.7 | 0.1 |
| Brick | 1 oz. | 105 | 8.4 | 5.3 | 0.0 | 0.8 | 0.1 |
| Brie | 1 oz. | 95 | 7.9 | 4.9 | 0.0 | 0.1 | 0.1 |
| Camembert | 1 oz. | 85 | 6.9 | 4.3 | 0.0 | 0.1 | 0.1 |
| Caraway | 1 oz. | 107 | 8.3 | 5.3 | 04 | 0.9 | n/a |
| Chavrie, goat's milk cheese | 2 tb. | 52 | 4.0 | 2.5 | 0.0 | 1.0 | 1.0 |
| Cheddar | 1 oz. | 114 | 9.4 | 6.0 | 0.0 | 0.4 | 0.2 |
| Alpine Lace, 50% less fat | 1 oz. | 70 | 4.5 | 3.0 | 0.0 | 1.0 | 0.0 |
| Cabot, light, 50% reduced fat | 1 oz. | 70 | 4.5 | 3.0 | 0.0 | 1.0 | 0.0 |
| ■ Lifeline, fat free | 1 oz. | 40 | 0.0 | 0.0 | 0.0 | 1.0 | 1.0 |
| ■ Fat & lactose free | 1 oz. | 40 | 0.0 | 0.0 | 0.0 | 1.0 | 1.0 |
| ■ Smart Beat lactose & fat free | 1 slice | 25 | 0.0 | 0.0 | 0.0 | 3.0 | 2.0 |
| Cheddar, shredded | | | | | | | |
| Cabot, light, shredded | ¼ cup | 70 | 4.5 | 3.0 | 0.0 | 1.0 | 0.0 |
| ■ Healthy Choice, fat free | ¼ cup | 45 | 0.0 | 0.0 | 0.0 | 2.0 | 0.0 |
| ■ Kraft Free | ¼ cup | 45 | 0.0 | 0.0 | 0.0 | 1.0 | 0.0 |
| Sharp, reduced fat | ¼ cup | 74 | 5.6 | 3.3 | 0.0 | 0.9 | 0.0 |
| Colby | 1 oz. | 112 | 9.1 | 5.7 | 0.0 | 0.7 | 0.2 |
| Cottage, small curd | ½ cup | 120 | 5.0 | 3.0 | 0.0 | 5.0 | 4.0 |
| ■ Low fat, low sodium | ½ cup | 81 | 1.1 | 0.7 | 0.0 | 3.0 | 3.0 |
| ■ Nonfat | ½ cup | 80 | 0.0 | 0.0 | 0.0 | 6.0 | 4.0 |
| Cream, Philadelphia, brick | 1 oz. | 100 | 10.0 | 6.0 | 0.0 | 1.0 | 1.0 |
| ■ Soft, fat free | 2 tb. | 30 | 0.0 | 0.0 | 0.0 | 2.0 | 1.0 |
| Soft, light | 2 tb. | 70 | 5.0 | 3.5 | 0.0 | 2.0 | 2.0 |
| Whipped | 2 tb. | 70 | 7.0 | 4.5 | 0.0 | 1.0 | 1.0 |
| Doux De Montagne | 1 oz. | 90 | 6.0 | 4.5 | 0.0 | 0.0 | 0.0 |
| Edam | 1 oz. | 101 | 7.9 | 5.0 | 0.0 | 0.4 | 0.4 |

■ Contains less than 20% fat
n/a Not available

| Item | SERVING | CAL-ORIES | FAT GRAMS | SAT. FAT GRAMS | TRANS FAT GRAMS | CARB. GRAMS | SUGAR GRAMS |
|---|---|---|---|---|---|---|---|
| Feta | 1 oz. | 60 | 4.5 | 3.0 | 0.0 | 1.0 | 0.0 |
| Alpine Lace, 50% less fat | 1 oz. | 50 | 3.0 | 2.0 | 0.0 | 1.0 | 0.0 |
| Fondue, Emmentaler | ¼ cup | 123 | 7.2 | 4.7 | 0.0 | 2.0 | n/a |
| Gorgonzola, crumbled | ¼ cup | 100 | 8.0 | 6.0 | 0.0 | 1.0 | 0.0 |
| Gouda | 1 oz. | 101 | 7.8 | 5.0 | 0.0 | 0.6 | 0.6 |
| Gruyere | 1 oz. | 117 | 9.2 | 5.4 | 0.0 | 0.1 | 0.1 |
| Havarti | 1 oz. | 122 | 10.1 | 7.1 | 0.0 | 0.0 | 0.0 |
| Light, Arla | 1 oz. | 80 | 4.0 | 3.0 | 0.0 | 0.0 | 0.0 |
| ■ Hickory smoked, Lifeline, fat free | 1 oz. | 40 | 0.0 | 0.0 | 0.0 | 1.0 | 1.0 |
| Jarlsberg Lite | 1 oz. | 70 | 3.5 | 2.0 | 0.0 | 0.0 | 0.0 |
| Mascarpone | 1 oz. | 126 | 13.2 | 7.1 | 0.0 | 1.0 | 0.0 |
| Limburger | 1 oz. | 93 | 7.7 | 4.8 | 0.0 | 0.1 | 0.1 |
| Monterey Jack | 1 oz. | 106 | 8.6 | 5.4 | 0.0 | 0.2 | 0.1 |
| Kraft, reduced fat | 1 oz. | 81 | 6.1 | 3.5 | 0.0 | 1.0 | 0.0 |
| Land O'Lakes, hot pepper | 1 oz. | 110 | 9.0 | 6.0 | 0.0 | 1.0 | 0.0 |
| ■ Lifeline, fat free | 1 oz. | 40 | 0.0 | 0.0 | 0.0 | 1.0 | 1.0 |
| Mozzarella | | | | | | | |
| Low moisture, part skim | 1 oz. | 70 | 4.0 | 3.0 | 2.0 | 1.0 | 0.0 |
| Shredded, Healthy Choice, reduced fat | ¼ cup | 70 | 4.0 | 2.5 | 0.0 | 1.0 | 0.0 |
| ■ Fat free | ¼ cup | 45 | 0.0 | 0.0 | 0.0 | 2.0 | 0.0 |
| String, Sargento, reduced fat | 1 each | 50 | 2.5 | 1.5 | 0.0 | 1.0 | 0.0 |
| Karoun, part skim | 1 oz. | 80 | 6.0 | 4.0 | 0.0 | 0.0 | 0.0 |
| Whole milk | 1 oz. | 85 | 6.3 | 3.7 | 0.0 | 0.6 | 0.3 |
| Muenster | 1 oz. | 104 | 8.5 | 5.4 | 0.0 | 0.3 | 0.3 |
| Neufchatel | 1 oz. | 74 | 6.6 | 4.2 | 0.0 | 0.8 | 0.3 |
| Old English, Kraft, sharp | 1 oz. | 80 | 7.1 | 4.4 | 0.0 | 0.9 | 0.0 |
| Parmesan, grated | 2 tsp. | 14 | 1.0 | 0.6 | 0.0 | 0.1 | 0.0 |
| Port De Salut | 1 oz. | 100 | 8.0 | 4.7 | 0.0 | 0.2 | 0.2 |
| Provolone | 1 oz. | 100 | 8.0 | 4.5 | 0.0 | 1.0 | 0.0 |
| Quark, fat-free, Appel Farms | ½ cup | 70 | 0.0 | 0.0 | 0.0 | 4.0 | 2.0 |
| Ricotta, whole milk | ¼ cup | 108 | 8.1 | 5.1 | 0.0 | 1.9 | 0.2 |
| Sargento, reduced fat | ¼ cup | 60 | 2.5 | 1.5 | 0.0 | 3.0 | 3.0 |
| Romano | 1 oz. | 110 | 7.6 | 4.9 | 0.0 | 1.0 | 0.2 |
| Roquefort | 1 oz. | 105 | 8.7 | 5.5 | 0.0 | 0.6 | n/a |
| Spread, American | 1 oz. | 82 | 6.0 | 3.8 | n/a | 2.5 | n/a |
| Boursin, Garlic & fine herbs | 2 tb. | 120 | 13.0 | 8.0 | 0.1 | <1 | n/a |
| Light | 2 tb. | 47 | 3.2 | 2.0 | 0.1 | <1 | n/a |
| Rondele, Garlic & fine herbs | 2 tb. | 70 | 7.0 | 5.0 | 0.1 | 1.0 | 1.0 |
| Light | 2 tb. | 50 | 4.0 | 2.5 | 0.1 | 2.0 | 1.0 |
| Cheese Whiz, Kraft | 2 tb. | 90 | 7.0 | 1.5 | 0.0 | 4.0 | 2.0 |
| Light | 1 oz. | 61 | 2.7 | 1.8 | 0.0 | 4.6 | 2.3 |
| Swiss | 1 oz. | 108 | 7.9 | 5.0 | 0.0 | 1.5 | 0.4 |
| Alpine Lace, 25% less fat, 53% less salt | 1 oz. | 90 | 6.0 | 4.0 | 0.0 | 1.0 | 0.0 |
| Kraft, reduced fat, slice | 1 slice | 97 | 6.7 | 4.5 | 0.0 | 0.8 | 0.0 |

■ Contains less than 20% fat

n/a Not available

| Item | SERVING | CAL-ORIES | FAT GRAMS | SAT. FAT GRAMS | TRANS FAT GRAMS | CARB. GRAMS | SUGAR GRAMS |
|---|---|---|---|---|---|---|---|
| ■ Lifeline, fat free | 1 oz. | 40 | 0.0 | 0.0 | 0.0 | 1.0 | 1.0 |
| Velveeta | 1 oz. | 80 | 6.0 | 3.5 | 0.0 | 3.0 | 2.0 |
| Light, reduced fat | 1 oz. | 63 | 3.0 | 2.0 | 0.0 | 3.4 | 2.4 |
| **Tofu (Soy) Cheeses** | | | | | | | |
| Cheddar substitute, Yves | 1 oz. | 50 | 2.8 | 0.0 | 0.0 | 1.4 | 0.0 |
| Cheese slices substitute, vegetarian, Veggie/Galaxy | 1 each | 40 | 2.0 | 0.0 | 0.0 | 1.0 | n/a |
| Cream cheese substitute, Toffuti | 1 oz. | 80 | 8.0 | 2.0 | 0.0 | 1.0 | 0.0 |
| Jalapeno Jack substitute, Yves | 1 oz. | 50 | 2.8 | 0.0 | 0.0 | 0.0 | 0.0 |
| Mozzarella substitute, Yves | 1 oz. | 43 | 2.8 | 0.0 | 0.0 | 0.0 | 0.0 |
| **Milk and Milk Beverages** | | | | | | | |
| Acidophilus 2% milk | 1 cup | 110 | 2.5 | 1.5 | 0.0 | 13.0 | 12.0 |
| ■ Nonfat/skim | 1 cup | 100 | 0.0 | 0.0 | 0.0 | 14.0 | 14.0 |
| ■ Buttermilk, skim | 1 cup | 90 | 0.0 | 0.0 | 0.0 | 13.0 | 12.0 |
| ■ Dry w/water added | 1 cup | 93 | 1.4 | 0.9 | 0.0 | 11.8 | n/a |
| ■ Low fat | 1 cup | 98 | 2.2 | 1.3 | 0.1 | 11.7 | 11.7 |
| Cream, half & half | 2 tb. | 39 | 3.5 | 2.2 | 0.1 | 1.3 | 0.1 |
| ■ Land O'Lakes, fat free | 2 tb. | 20 | 0.0 | 0.0 | 0.0 | 3.0 | 2.0 |
| Cream, heavy | | | | | | | |
| Unwhipped | 2 tb. | 103 | 11.0 | 6.9 | 0.3 | 0.8 | 0.0 |
| Whipped | 2 tb. | 52 | 5.5 | 3.4 | 0.2 | 0.4 | 0.0 |
| Cream, light (whipping) | | | | | | | |
| Unwhipped | 2 tb. | 87 | 9.2 | 5.8 | 0.3 | 0.9 | 0.0 |
| Whipped | 2 tb. | 44 | 4.6 | 2.9 | 0.1 | 0.4 | 0.0 |
| Cream, sour | 2 tb. | 62 | 6.0 | 3.8 | 0.2 | 1.2 | 0.1 |
| Knudsen, light | 2 tb. | 40 | 2.5 | 2.0 | 0.0 | 2.0 | 2.0 |
| ■ Fat free | 2 tb. | 35 | 0.0 | 0.0 | 0.0 | 6.0 | 2.0 |
| Land O'Lakes | 2 tb. | 35 | 2.0 | 1.5 | 0.0 | 4.0 | 2.0 |
| ■ Nonfat | 2 tb. | 30 | 0.0 | 0.0 | 0.0 | 5.0 | 2.0 |
| Cream, sour, imitation, Imo | 2 tb. | 60 | 5.0 | 5.0 | 0.0 | 2.0 | 2.0 |
| Creamer, nondairy, Coffee Rich | 1 tb. | 18 | 1.2 | 0.3 | n/a | 1.8 | 0.5 |
| Coffee Mate | 1 tb. | 10 | 0.5 | 0.5 | 0.0 | 1.0 | 0.0 |
| Dry Original | 1 tsp. | 10 | 0.5 | 0.5 | 0.0 | 1.0 | 0.0 |
| ■ Fat free | 1 tb. | 10 | 0.0 | 0.0 | 0.0 | 2.0 | 0.0 |
| Hazelnut, sugar free | 1 tb. | 30 | 2.5 | 2.0 | 0.0 | 2.0 | 0.0 |
| ■ Mocha, fat free | 1 tb. | 25 | 0.0 | 0.0 | 0.0 | 5.0 | 5.0 |
| Condensed, sweetened, canned, Eagle | 2 tb. | 120 | 1.5 | 1.0 | 0.0 | 23.0 | 23.0 |
| Eggnog, nonalcoholic | 1 cup | 400 | 18.0 | 10.0 | 0.0 | 50.0 | 48.0 |
| Evaporated, whole, Carnation | 1 cup | 320 | 16.0 | 12.0 | 0.0 | 24.0 | 24.0 |
| ■ Low fat | 1 cup | 200 | 4.0 | 4.0 | 0.0 | 24.0 | 24.0 |
| ■ Nonfat/skim | 1 cup | 200 | 0.0 | 0.0 | 0.0 | 32.0 | 32.0 |
| Hot cocoa, prepared w/whole milk | 1 cup | 213 | 8.3 | 5.2 | n/a | 29.4 | n/a |
| ■ Carnation, fat free, dry | 1 packet | 25 | 0.0 | 0.0 | 0.0 | 4.0 | 3.0 |

■ Contains less than 20% fat
n/a Not available

| Item | SERVING | CAL-ORIES | FAT GRAMS | SAT. FAT GRAMS | TRANS FAT GRAMS | CARB. GRAMS | SUGAR GRAMS |
|---|---|---|---|---|---|---|---|
| ■ w/marshmallows | I each | 40 | 0.0 | 0.0 | 0.0 | 8.0 | 6.0 |
| Swiss Miss, dry | I packet | 120 | 3.0 | 1.0 | 0.0 | 22.0 | 17.0 |
| ■ Diet, w/calcium | I packet | 25 | 0.0 | 0.0 | 0.0 | 4.0 | 2.0 |
| ■ Fat free | I packet | 50 | 0.0 | 0.0 | 0.0 | 9.0 | 9.0 |
| ■ Sugar free, dry | I packet | 50 | 1.0 | 0.0 | 0.0 | 10.0 | 7.0 |
| ■ Marshmallows w/calcium | I packet | 60 | 1.0 | 0.0 | 0.0 | 10.0 | 7.0 |
| Lactaid, low fat 1% milk | 8 oz. | 110 | 2.5 | 1.5 | 0.0 | 13.0 | 12.0 |
| ■ Fat free | 8 oz. | 80 | 0.0 | 0.0 | 0.0 | 13.0 | 12.0 |
| Milk, chocolate | I cup | 208 | 8.5 | 5.3 | 0.3 | 25.9 | 23.9 |
| ■ Low fat | 8 oz. | 150 | 2.5 | 1.5 | 0.0 | 26.0 | 25.0 |
| ■ Nonfat/skim | I cup | 144 | 1.2 | 0.7 | 0.0 | 26.7 | 22.8 |
| 2% | I cup | 180 | 5.0 | 3.1 | 0.2 | 26.0 | 24.8 |
| Milk, whole, 3.3% fat | I cup | 146 | 7.9 | 4.6 | 0.2 | 11.0 | 11.0 |
| 2% fat | I cup | 122 | 4.8 | 3.1 | 0.2 | 11.4 | 11.4 |
| 2% Parmalat, shelf stable | I cup | 130 | 5.0 | 3.0 | 0.0 | 12.0 | 12.0 |
| 1% fat | I cup | 102 | 2.4 | 1.5 | 0.1 | 12.2 | 12.2 |
| ■ Nonfat/skim | I cup | 90 | 0.0 | 0.0 | 0.0 | 13.0 | 12.0 |
| Milk, whole, dry | ¼ cup | 159 | 8.6 | 5.4 | 0.3 | 12.3 | 12.3 |
| ■ Nonfat/skim, dry | ¼ cup | 61 | 0.0 | 0.0 | 0.0 | 9.1 | 9.1 |
| Milk, goat | I cup | 168 | 10.1 | 6.5 | 0.0 | 10.9 | 10.9 |
| Milk, malted, chocolate, w/whole milk | I cup | 225 | 8.7 | 5.0 | n/a | 29.7 | 17.7 |
| ■ w/skim milk | I cup | 146 | 1.1 | 0.7 | 0.0 | 27.0 | n/a |
| Milk shake, chocolate | I cup | 211 | 6.2 | 3.9 | 0.0 | 34.1 | 31.0 |
| Vanilla | I cup | 185 | 5.0 | 3.1 | 0.0 | 29.8 | 29.6 |
| Nesquik chocolate | 8 oz. | 193 | 6.7 | 4.2 | 0.0 | 27.7 | 25.2 |
| ■ Fat free | 8 oz. | 143 | 0.0 | 0.0 | 0.0 | 27.7 | 25.9 |
| Strawberry | 8 oz. | 194 | 6.8 | 4.2 | 0.0 | 27.8 | 25.3 |
| **Nondairy Milk Beverages** | | | | | | | |
| ■ Rice Dream, original | I cup | 120 | 2.0 | 0.0 | 0.0 | 25.0 | 11.0 |
| ■ Vanilla | I cup | 130 | 2.0 | 0.0 | 0.0 | 28.0 | 12.0 |
| Soy milk, Eden, original | I cup | 130 | 4.0 | 0.5 | 0.0 | 13.0 | 7.0 |
| ■ Vanilla | I cup | 150 | 3.0 | 0.0 | 0.0 | 23.0 | 15.0 |
| Vitasoy, original, light | I cup | 90 | 2.0 | 0.0 | 0.0 | 15.0 | n/a |
| ■ WestSoy, Vanilla Lite | 8 oz. | 120 | 2.5 | 0.5 | 0.0 | 21.0 | 15.0 |
| **Yogurt** | | | | | | | |
| Dairy | | | | | | | |
| Yogurt, plain, whole | 8 oz. | 138 | 7.4 | 4.8 | 0.0 | 10.6 | 10.6 |
| Low fat | 8 oz. | 143 | 3.5 | 2.3 | 0.0 | 16.0 | 16.0 |
| ■ Fage, plain, nonfat Greek | 5.3 oz. | 80 | 0.0 | 0.0 | 0.0 | 6.0 | 6.0 |
| ■ Dannon, blueberry, nonfat, light, w/aspartame | 8 oz. | 120 | 0.0 | 0.0 | 0.0 | 23.0 | 17.0 |
| ■ Cherry Vanilla Light and Fit | 6 oz. | 90 | 0.0 | 0.0 | 0.0 | 16.0 | 12.0 |
| ■ Lemon Meringue Pie, low fat | 8 oz. | 240 | 1.3 | 0.7 | 0.0 | 49.4 | 44.0 |

■ Contains less than 20% fat
n/a Not available

19

| Item | SERVING | CAL-ORIES | FAT GRAMS | SAT. FAT GRAMS | TRANS FAT GRAMS | CARB. GRAMS | SUGAR GRAMS |
|---|---|---|---|---|---|---|---|
| ■ Strawberry banana, Fruit on the Bottom | 8 oz. | 210 | 2.0 | 1.0 | 0.0 | 40.0 | 34.0 |
| ■ Vanilla, nonfat, light, w/aspartame | 8 oz. | 120 | 0.0 | 0.0 | 0.0 | 21.0 | 15.0 |
| ■ Yoplait, Healthy Heart (Plant Sterols) | 6 oz. | 180 | 1.5 | 0.5 | 0.0 | 35.0 | 27.0 |
| ■ Light, fat free, strawberry | 6 oz. | 100 | 0.0 | 0.0 | 0.0 | 19.0 | 14.0 |

**Nondairy Yogurt**

| Item | SERVING | CAL-ORIES | FAT GRAMS | SAT. FAT GRAMS | TRANS FAT GRAMS | CARB. GRAMS | SUGAR GRAMS |
|---|---|---|---|---|---|---|---|
| ■ Soy, Silk, vanilla | 1 each | 120 | 2.0 | 0.0 | 0.0 | 23.0 | 16.0 |

# DESSERTS

**Cakes**

| Item | SERVING | CAL-ORIES | FAT GRAMS | SAT. FAT GRAMS | TRANS FAT GRAMS | CARB. GRAMS | SUGAR GRAMS |
|---|---|---|---|---|---|---|---|
| ■ Angel Food, from mix, Gold Medal | 1 piece | 120 | 0.0 | 0.0 | 0.0 | 27.0 | 20.0 |
| Banana, Sara Lee | 1/5 cake | 280 | 10.0 | 3.5 | 1.0 | 46.0 | 34.0 |
| Black Forest | 2 oz. | 198 | 10.9 | n/a | n/a | 23.0 | 17.0 |
| ■ Brownie, low fat, from mix, Betty Crocker | 1/18 package | 130 | 2.5 | <1 | n/a | 27.0 | 18.0 |
| Butter Loaf, Entenmann's | 1 piece | 280 | 15.0 | 3.5 | n/a | 36.0 | 27.0 |
| Carrot, Mrs. Smith's | 1 piece | 300 | 16.0 | 4.0 | 1.5 | 37.0 | 27.0 |
| Gold Medal, from mix | 1 piece | 210 | 12.0 | 2.5 | n/a | 24.0 | 14.0 |
| * Cheesecake, homemade | 2 oz. | 182 | 12.8 | 5.6 | n/a | 14.5 | n/a |
| ■ Fat free | 2 oz. | 87 | 0.0 | 0.0 | 0.0 | 18.0 | 11.3 |
| ■ Gold Medal, plain, from mix | 1 piece | 70 | 1.5 | 0.5 | n/a | 12.0 | 10.0 |
| Jell-O No Bake, strawberry, from mix | 1 piece | 340 | 12.0 | 4.5 | 0.0 | 52.0 | 36.0 |
| Reduced fat | 1 piece | 250 | 6.0 | 2.0 | 0.0 | 44.0 | 33.0 |
| ■ Krusteaz, lemon, fat free, frozen | 2 oz. | 100 | 0.1 | 0.0 | 0.0 | 20.4 | 14.7 |
| Sara Lee, original, frozen | 1/4 cake | 330 | 17.0 | 8.0 | 1.5 | 35.0 | 24.0 |
| *■ Chocolate, homemade | 2 oz. | 208 | 9.3 | 2.7 | n/a | 31.0 | n/a |
| Gold Medal, from mix | 1 piece | 200 | 10.0 | 2.5 | n/a | 26.0 | 16.0 |
| Chocolate fudge, layer, Pepperidge Farm | 1 piece | 300 | 16.0 | 5.0 | 3.5 | 38.0 | 18.0 |
| Coconut layer, Mrs. Smiths | 1 piece | 350 | 20.0 | 7.0 | 0.0 | 41.0 | 33.0 |
| * Coffee, homemade | 2 oz. | 180 | 5.4 | 1.1 | n/a | 29.9 | 16.7 |
| Koffee Kake, juniors, TastyKake | 1 | 270 | 9.0 | 1.5 | n/a | 43.0 | 22.0 |
| Cupcake, chocolate, homemade, w/egg/milk | 2 oz. | 198 | 6.8 | 0.5 | n/a | 28.9 | n/a |
| Hostess | 1 | 180 | 6.0 | 2.5 | 0.0 | 30.0 | 17.0 |
| ■ Light | 1 | 130 | 1.0 | 0.0 | 0.0 | 30.0 | 22.0 |
| Little Debbie, creme filled | 1 | 200 | 10.0 | 2.5 | 3.0 | 26.0 | 18.0 |
| TastyKake | 1 | 110 | 3.0 | 0.8 | n/a | 19.5 | 12.0 |
| Devil Cakes, Little Debbie | 2 | 280 | 13.0 | 3.0 | 5.0 | 39.0 | 26.0 |
| Devil Dog, Drakes | 1 | 180 | 8.0 | 2.0 | 2.0 | 26.0 | 16.0 |

| Item | SERVING | CAL-ORIES | FAT GRAMS | SAT. FAT GRAMS | TRANS FAT GRAMS | CARB. GRAMS | SUGAR GRAMS |
|---|---|---|---|---|---|---|---|
| Reduced fat | 1 | 160 | 4.0 | 1.0 | 1.0 | 29.0 | 18.0 |
| Devils Food, from mix, Gold Medal | 2 oz. | 268 | 12.7 | 3.8 | 3.0 | 31.9 | 20.4 |
| Pepperidge Farm, layer | 2 oz. | 206 | 9.9 | 3.5 | n/a | 28.4 | 12.8 |
| Ding Dongs, Hostess | 1 | 350 | 18.0 | 13.0 | 0.0 | 47.0 | 37.0 |
| * ■ Fruitcake, homemade | 2 oz. | 184 | 5.2 | 0.6 | n/a | 34.9 | 15.6 |
| German chocolate layer, Pepperidge Farm | 1 piece | 300 | 16.0 | 4.0 | 3.0 | 37.0 | 18.0 |
| Gingerbread, from mix, Gold Medal | 2 oz. | 240 | 5.6 | 1.6 | n/a | 41.6 | 16.0 |
| Golden layer, Pepperidge Farm | 1 piece | 290 | 14.0 | 3.0 | n/a | 40.0 | n/a |
| Ho Hos, Hostess | 2 | 250 | 12.0 | 8.0 | 0.2 | 34.0 | 23.0 |
| Icing/frosting | | | | | | | |
| Coconut pecan, Betty Crocker | 1 oz. | 140 | 7.0 | 3.0 | 1.5 | 18.0 | 15.0 |
| * Chocolate | 1 oz. | 140 | 5.0 | 2.0 | 1.5 | 18.0 | 16.0 |
| Chocolate fudge | 1 oz. | 140 | 5.1 | 1.8 | 2.0 | 17.6 | 15.6 |
| Cream cheese, Betty Crocker | 1 oz. | 122 | 4.9 | 1.2 | 2.0 | 19.4 | 17.8 |
| Vanilla creme, Gold Medal | 1 oz. | 120 | 4.3 | 1.1 | 2.0 | 20.4 | 19.0 |
| White cream, Krusteaz, from mix | 1 oz. | 122 | 5.1 | 0.8 | n/a | 18.2 | 16.2 |
| Lemon, layer, Mrs. Smith's | 1 piece | 290 | 12.0 | 3.5 | n/a | 43.0 | 32.0 |
| Marble, w/chocolate icing, homemade | 2 oz. | 193 | 7.1 | 2.8 | n/a | 31.3 | 22.9 |
| Oatmeal creme pies, Little Debbie | 1 | 170 | 7.0 | 1.5 | 2.0 | 26.0 | 14.0 |
| * Pineapple upside down, homemade | 2 oz. | 181 | 6.9 | 1.7 | 0.0 | 28.6 | n/a |
| Pound, gold, from mix, Gold Medal | 2 oz. | 289 | 13.1 | 3.9 | n/a | 36.8 | 26.3 |
| Pound cake, Sara Lee, butter | ¼ cake | 300 | 16.0 | 8.0 | 1.0 | 35.0 | 20.0 |
| Ring Dings | 2 | 340 | 18.0 | 7.0 | 2.0 | 43.0 | 30.0 |
| Sno Balls, Hostess | 1 | 170 | 5.0 | 3.5 | 0.0 | 32.0 | 24.0 |
| Spice, from mix, Gold Medal | 2 oz. | 255 | 12.7 | 5.4 | n/a | 33.1 | 20.4 |
| ■ Sponge, homemade | 1 piece | 187 | 2.7 | 0.8 | 0.0 | 36.4 | n/a |
| Shortcake, strawberry, Sara Lee | ⅛ cake | 180 | 7.0 | 4.5 | 3.0 | 27.0 | 16.0 |
| Swiss Cake Rolls, Little Debbie | 2 | 270 | 12.0 | 3.0 | 4.5 | 38.0 | 25.0 |
| Twinkie, Hostess | 1 | 150 | 5.0 | 1.5 | 0.0 | 25.0 | 14.0 |
| ■ Light | 1 | 120 | 1.0 | 0.0 | 0.0 | 28.0 | 17.0 |
| White, w/chocolate icing, homemade | 2 oz. | 243 | 8.1 | 4.1 | n/a | 42.8 | 37.8 |
| Yellow, w/chocolate icing | 2 oz. | 215 | 9.9 | 2.6 | n/a | 31.4 | n/a |
| ■ Yellow, from mix, Betty Crocker | 1/12 cake | 250 | 2.5 | 1.0 | 0.0 | 36.0 | 22.0 |
| Gold Medal, from mix | 2 oz. | 255 | 11.5 | 3.2 | n/a | 33.1 | 20.4 |
| ■ Zebra Cakes, Little Debbie | 2 | 270 | 13.0 | 3.0 | 4.0 | 37.0 | 30.0 |

---

■ Contains less than 20% fat
n/a Not available

* See note, page xli

| Item | SERVING | CAL-ORIES | FAT GRAMS | SAT. FAT GRAMS | TRANS FAT GRAMS | CARB. GRAMS | SUGAR GRAMS |
|---|---|---|---|---|---|---|---|
| **Pies** | | | | | | | |
| Apple, homemade | 1 piece | 411 | 19.4 | 4.7 | n/a | 57.5 | n/a |
| Mrs. Smith's | 1 piece | 350 | 14.0 | 3.0 | 4.0 | 55.0 | 30.0 |
| No sugar added | 1 piece | 350 | 20.0 | 4.0 | 0.0 | 42.0 | 8.0 |
| Reduced fat | 1 piece | 230 | 8.0 | 2.0 | 0.0 | 41.0 | 14.0 |
| Banana cream, Claim Jumper | 3.5 oz. | 290 | 17.0 | 8.0 | 2.0 | 30.0 | 18.0 |
| Blackberry cobbler | 4 oz. | 240 | 8.0 | 3.5 | 0.0 | 42.0 | 23.0 |
| * ■ Blueberry cobbler | 3 oz. | 208 | 10.1 | 2.5 | n/a | 28.5 | n/a |
| Boston cream | 3 oz. | 214 | 7.2 | 2.1 | n/a | 36.5 | 30.7 |
| Cherry, Sara Lee | 4.5 oz. | 340 | 16.0 | 7.0 | 0.0 | 45.0 | 14.0 |
| Chocolate Silk | 3.5 oz. | 410 | 30.0 | 13.0 | 5.0 | 36.0 | 25.0 |
| Chocolate Meringue, Mrs. Smith's | 3 oz. | 198 | 7.8 | 2.8 | n/a | 30.5 | 22.0 |
| Coconut cream, Claim Jumper | 3.8 oz. | 310 | 18.0 | 10.0 | 2.0 | 32.0 | 20.0 |
| Coconut custard, Mrs. Smith's | 3 oz. | 184 | 9.5 | 3.4 | n/a | 20.4 | 11.6 |
| Key lime | 4.5 oz. | 450 | 22.0 | 15.0 | 1.5 | 58.0 | 47.0 |
| Lemon meringue, Mrs. Smith's | 3 oz. | 177 | 4.3 | 1.1 | n/a | 32.6 | 23.4 |
| Mincemeat, Homemade | 3 oz. | 246 | 9.2 | 2.3 | n/a | 40.8 | 24.1 |
| Mrs. Smith's | 1/8 pie | 380 | 17.0 | 3.5 | n/a | 53.0 | 26.0 |
| Peach lattice, Mrs. Smith's | 3 oz. | 191 | 8.5 | 1.8 | 0.0 | 26.9 | 11.3 |
| Peach, reduced fat, Mrs. Smith's | 3 oz. | 153 | 5.6 | 1.4 | 0.0 | 26.5 | 7.0 |
| Pecan, Mrs. Smith's | 3 oz. | 365 | 17.3 | 4.0 | n/a | 49.8 | 29.2 |
| Pumpkin, Mrs. Smith's | 3 oz. | 211 | 8.2 | 2.0 | 0.0 | 32.0 | 17.7 |
| Sour cream raisin | 3 oz. | 309 | 20.0 | 7.2 | n/a | 29.5 | n/a |
| Rhubarb | 3 oz. | 228 | 9.4 | 2.6 | n/a | 34.5 | 19.5 |
| Strawberries and creme, Sara Lee | 1/8 pie | 350 | 20.0 | 12.0 | 2.0 | 42.0 | 22.0 |
| Sweet potato, Mrs. Smith's | 3 oz. | 259 | 10.6 | 3.3 | n/a | 37.2 | 23.3 |
| * ■ Tart, apple, w/apricot glaze | 1 | 147 | 0.7 | 0.1 | 0.0 | 0.0 | n/a |
| * ■ Yogurt, lemon-lime | 1 serv. | 84 | 1.2 | 0.5 | 0.0 | 0.0 | n/a |
| | | | | | | | |
| **Pie Crusts & Fillings** | | | | | | | |
| Pie crusts | | | | | | | |
| Chocolate, Ready Crust, Keebler | 1/8 | 87 | 4.0 | 0.9 | 1.5 | 12.2 | 5.8 |
| Graham, Ready Crust, Keebler | 1/8 | 89 | 4.3 | 0.9 | 2.0 | 11.9 | 4.9 |
| Reduced fat | 1/8 crust | 90 | 3.5 | 0.5 | 1.5 | 15.0 | 6.0 |
| Deep dish, 9", Mrs. Smith's | 1/8 | 150 | 10.0 | 2.0 | 0.0 | 14.0 | n/a |
| Pie crust from mix | 1/8 | 100 | 6.1 | 1.5 | n/a | 10.1 | n/a |
| Pillsbury Just Unroll Pie Crust, Refrigerated | 1/8 | 120 | 7.0 | 2.5 | 2.5 | 13.0 | 1.0 |
| Puff Pastry Sheets, Pepperidge Farm | 1/6 sheet | 200 | 11.0 | 2.5 | 4.0 | 23.0 | 0.0 |
| Pie Filling | | | | | | | |
| ■ Apple, More Fruit, Comstock/ Wilderness | 1/3 cup | 80 | 0.0 | 0.0 | 0.0 | 20.0 | 18.0 |

■ Contains less than 20% fat
n/a Not available

* See note, page xli

| Item | SERVING | CAL-ORIES | FAT GRAMS | SAT. FAT GRAMS | TRANS FAT GRAMS | CARB. GRAMS | SUGAR GRAMS |
|---|---|---|---|---|---|---|---|
| ■ Butterscotch, fat & sugar free, Jell-O | ¼ package | 70 | 0.0 | 0.0 | 0.0 | 6.0 | 0.0 |
| ■ Cherry, Red Ruby original, Comstock/Wilderness | ⅓ cup | 90 | 0.0 | 0.0 | 0.0 | 23.0 | 19.0 |
| ■ Chocolate, Jell-O | ¼ package | 160 | 0.0 | 0.0 | 0.0 | 25.0 | 19.0 |
| ■ Chocolate, fat & sugar free, Jell-O | ¼ | 80 | 0.0 | 0.0 | 0.0 | 8.0 | 0.0 |
| ■ Lemon, Jell-O | ¼ package | 150 | 0.0 | 0.0 | 0.0 | 24.0 | 19.0 |

**Puddings**

| Item | SERVING | CAL-ORIES | FAT GRAMS | SAT. FAT GRAMS | TRANS FAT GRAMS | CARB. GRAMS | SUGAR GRAMS |
|---|---|---|---|---|---|---|---|
| * Bread | 3 oz. | 149 | 5.3 | 2.5 | n/a | 20.8 | 12.7 |
| * ■ Raisin bread | ½ cup | 74 | 0.5 | 0.1 | 0.0 | n/a | n/a |
| ■ Chocolate, from mix, Jell-O | ½ cup | 150 | 2.5 | 1.5 | 0.0 | 28.0 | 21.0 |
| ■ Fat free | ½ cup | 130 | 0.0 | 0.0 | 0.0 | 29.0 | 21.0 |
| Snack cup, Jell-O | 1 | 160 | 5.0 | 2.0 | 0.0 | 28.0 | 23.0 |
| ■ Fat free | 1 | 102 | 0.5 | 0.3 | 0.0 | 22.7 | 17.3 |
| Chocolate Vanilla Swirl, snack cup, Jell-O | 1 | 160 | 5.0 | 2.0 | 0.0 | 27.0 | 22.0 |
| ■ Fat free | 1 | 100 | 0.0 | 0.0 | 0.0 | 23.0 | 17.0 |
| ■ Devil's food, fat free, snack cup, Jell-O | 1 | 100 | 0.0 | 0.0 | 0.0 | 23.0 | 18.0 |
| Egg custard, snack cup, Swiss Miss | 1 | 140 | 5.0 | 2.0 | 0.0 | 19.0 | 16.0 |
| ■ Lemon, from mix, Jell-O | ½ cup | 140 | 2.0 | 0.5 | 0.0 | 29.0 | 23.0 |
| ■ Pistachio, instant from mix, Jell-O | ½ cup | 160 | 3.0 | 1.5 | 0.0 | 29.0 | 24.0 |
| ■ Rice, raisin, Lundberg Farms | 1 serv. | 64 | 0.0 | 0.0 | 0.0 | 14.6 | 6.4 |
| ■ Rocky Road, fat free, snack cup, Jell-O | 1 | 100 | 0.0 | 0.0 | 0.0 | 23.0 | 17.0 |
| Tapioca, snack cup, Jell-O | 1 | 140 | 4.0 | 1.5 | 0.0 | 26.0 | 21.0 |
| ■ Fat free | 1 | 100 | 0.0 | 0.0 | 0.0 | 23.0 | 17.0 |
| ■ Vanilla, from mix, Jell-O | ½ cup | 140 | 2.5 | 1.5 | 0.0 | 26.0 | 21.0 |
| ■ Fat free | ½ cup | 140 | 0.0 | 0.0 | 0.0 | 29.0 | 25.0 |
| Snack cup, Jell-O | 1 | 160 | 5.0 | 2.0 | 0.0 | 25.0 | 21.0 |
| ■ Fat free | 1 | 104 | 0.2 | 0.2 | 0.0 | 23.2 | 17.9 |

**Other Desserts**

| Item | SERVING | CAL-ORIES | FAT GRAMS | SAT. FAT GRAMS | TRANS FAT GRAMS | CARB. GRAMS | SUGAR GRAMS |
|---|---|---|---|---|---|---|---|
| Baklava, homemade | 1 oz. | 122 | 8.3 | 3.4 | n/a | 10.7 | n/a |
| Cobbler, peach, Mrs. Smith's | 4 oz. | 240 | 8.0 | 3.5 | 0.0 | 40.0 | 22.0 |
| Light | 2 oz. | 120 | 2.7 | 1.7 | 0.0 | 20.0 | 11.0 |
| * ■ Cobbler, blueberry meringue | 1 serv. | 127 | 0.3 | 0.0 | n/a | n/a | n/a |
| Cream puff, custard filled, profiteroles | 1 | 280 | 22 | 14 | 0.5 | 17.0 | 11.0 |
| Dumpling, apple, frozen, Pepperidge Farm | 1 | 290 | 11.0 | 2.5 | n/a | 44.0 | 6.0 |
| Eclair, chocolate, Smart Ones | 1 | 150 | 4.0 | 1.0 | 0.0 | 25.0 | 13.0 |
| Jell-O gelatin, from mix | | | | | | | |
| ■ Cherry | ½ cup | 80 | 0.0 | 0.0 | 0.0 | 19.0 | 19.0 |

| Item | SERVING | CAL-ORIES | FAT GRAMS | SAT. FAT GRAMS | TRANS FAT GRAMS | CARB. GRAMS | SUGAR GRAMS |
|---|---|---|---|---|---|---|---|
| ■     Sugar free | ½ cup | 10 | 0.0 | 0.0 | 0.0 | 0.0 | 0.0 |
| ■   Lime | ½ cup | 80 | 0.0 | 0.0 | 0.0 | 19.0 | 19.0 |
| Mousse, chocolate, Smart Ones | 1 serv. | 180 | 4.0 | 3.0 | 0.0 | 24.0 | 12.0 |
| Strudel, apple, Trader Joe's | 3" slice | 300 | 17.0 | 6.0 | 0.0 | 32.0 | 13.0 |
| * ■ Trifle, chocolate | 1 serv. | 69 | 1.5 | 0.2 | 0.0 | n/a | n/a |
| Turnover, apple, Pepperidge Farm, frozen | 1 | 284 | 16.0 | 4.0 | 5.0 | 31.2 | 10.8 |

**Toppings**

| Item | SERVING | CAL-ORIES | FAT GRAMS | SAT. FAT GRAMS | TRANS FAT GRAMS | CARB. GRAMS | SUGAR GRAMS |
|---|---|---|---|---|---|---|---|
| ■ Butterscotch | 2 tb. | 103 | 0.0 | 0.0 | 0.0 | 27.0 | n/a |
| ■ Caramel, fat free, Smucker's | 2 tb. | 110 | 0.0 | 0.0 | 0.0 | 28.0 | 28.0 |
| ■ Cherry | 2 tb. | 98 | 0.0 | 0.0 | 0.0 | 24.4 | 10.7 |
| Chocolate, fudge, Hershey's | 2 tb. | 140 | 6.0 | 4.0 | 0.0 | 20.0 | n/a |
| Hot fudge | 2 tb. | 140 | 4.5 | 2.0 | 0.0 | 24.0 | 17.0 |
| ■ Fat free, Hershey's | 2 tb. | 100 | 0.0 | 0.0 | 0.0 | 23.0 | n/a |
| ■ Smucker's | 2 tb. | 100 | 0.0 | 0.0 | 0.0 | 26.0 | 16.0 |
| ■ Sauce, fruit sweetened, Orchard Farms | 2 tb. | 90 | 0.5 | 0.0 | 0.0 | 21.0 | 18.0 |
| Sauce, Scharffen Berger | 2 tb. | 120 | 6.0 | 4.0 | 0.0 | 15.0 | 12.0 |
| ■ Syrup, Hershey's | 2 tb. | 100 | 0.0 | 0.0 | 0.0 | 24.0 | 20.0 |
| ■ Light | 2 tb. | 50 | 0.2 | 0.0 | 0.0 | 11.9 | 10.0 |
| Cool Whip, nondairy | 2 tb. | 25 | 1.5 | 1.5 | 0.0 | 2.0 | 1.0 |
| Extra Creamy | 2 tb. | 25 | 2.0 | 2.0 | 0.0 | 2.0 | 1.0 |
| Light, Cool Whip | 2 tb. | 20 | 1.0 | 1.0 | 0.0 | 2.0 | 1.0 |
| ■ Fat free | 2 tb. | 15 | 0.0 | 0.0 | 0.0 | 3.0 | 1.0 |
| ■ Marshmallow creme | 2 tb. | 40 | 0.0 | 0.0 | 0.0 | 10.0 | 8.0 |
| Raisin sauce | 2 tb. | 40 | 1.6 | 0.3 | 0.0 | 6.8 | n/a |
| ■ Strawberry, Smucker's | 2 tb. | 100 | 0.0 | 0.0 | 0.0 | 26.0 | 26.0 |
| Whipped topping, nondairy from can | 2 tb. | 23 | 2.0 | 1.7 | 0.0 | 1.4 | 1.4 |
| Fat free, Reddi-wip | ½ oz. | 21 | 0.7 | 0.4 | 0.0 | 3.5 | 2.3 |

## DINING OUT

Restaurants are **not required** to provide a nutritional analysis. Moreover, different restaurants use different recipes in the preparation of their foods. Ask when eating out or ordering in which fats are being used in food preparation.

**Chinese**
Beef

| Item | SERVING | CAL-ORIES | FAT GRAMS | SAT. FAT GRAMS | TRANS FAT GRAMS | CARB. GRAMS | SUGAR GRAMS |
|---|---|---|---|---|---|---|---|
| w/broccoli | 1 each | 350 | 10.0 | 5.0 | n/a | 53.0 | 25.0 |
| Szechuan style w/lo mein & vegetables | 1.5 cup | 476 | 20.0 | 7.0 | n/a | 40.0 | n/a |
| w/sweet & sour | 1 cup | 336 | 18.1 | 6.1 | n/a | 27.8 | n/a |
| ■ Buns, Chinese steamed | 1 each | 90 | 1.0 | 0.0 | 0.0 | 18.0 | 1.5 |
| Chicken, skinned and boneless w/black bean sauce | 4 oz. chicken | 480 | 27.0 | n/a | n/a | n/a | n/a |

---

■ Contains less than 20% fat
n/a Not available

* See note, page xli

| Item | SERVING | CAL-ORIES | FAT GRAMS | SAT. FAT GRAMS | TRANS FAT GRAMS | CARB. GRAMS | SUGAR GRAMS |
|---|---|---|---|---|---|---|---|
| Chicken, w/cashew nuts or walnuts | 1 cup | 431 | 31.0 | 5.0 | n/a | 11.0 | n/a |
| Chicken, kung pao, white meat | 1 cup | 431 | 30.6 | 5.2 | n/a | 11.4 | n/a |
| Cookie, almond | 1 each | 52 | 3.2 | 0.5 | n/a | 5.2 | 2.4 |
| ■ Cookie, fortune | 1 each | 30 | 0.2 | 0.1 | 0.0 | 6.7 | 3.6 |
| Duck, white Peking, breast, w/skin | 4 oz. | 229 | 12.3 | 3.3 | n/a | 0.0 | 0.0 |
| Dumplings (pot stickers), fried, chicken | 2 pieces | 44 | 2.0 | 0.6 | 0.0 | 3.8 | 0.4 |
| Pork | 2 pieces | 49 | 2.2 | 0.9 | 0.0 | 4.7 | 0.2 |
| Shrimp | 2 pieces | 47 | 2.2 | 0.4 | 0.0 | 4.2 | 0.4 |
| Egg roll, shrimp | 1 each | 104 | 5.6 | 1.2 | n/a | 9.9 | n/a |
| Fish | | | | | | | |
| ■ Salmon, sweet and sour | 3 oz. | 197 | 4.0 | n/a | 0.0 | 16.0 | n/a |
| ■ Snapper, steamed | 3 oz. | 109 | 1.5 | 0.3 | 0.0 | 0.0 | 0.0 |
| Lo mein, vegetable | 5.5 oz. | 205 | 5.5 | 1.5 | 0.0 | 30.0 | 3.0 |
| * Pork | | | | | | | |
| Barbecued | 4 oz. | 204 | 10.0 | 4.0 | 0.0 | 3.0 | n/a |
| Sweet & sour | 1 cup | 231 | 8.3 | 2.1 | 0.0 | 25.1 | 19.1 |
| Rice, fried | 1 cup | 271 | 12.4 | 1.8 | 0.0 | 34.2 | 1.0 |
| Shellfish | | | | | | | |
| Crab w/black bean sauce | 12–16 oz. | 325 | 24.0 | n/a | 0.0 | n/a | 0.0 |
| Crab Rangoon | 1 | 70 | 6.0 | n/a | n/a | 3.0 | n/a |
| Lobster Cantonese | 6 oz. in shell | 295 | 17.0 | n/a | n/a | n/a | n/a |
| Shrimp, sweet and sour | 4 oz. shrimp | 213 | 9.0 | 2.0 | n/a | 3.0 | n/a |
| Shrimp, w/lobster sauce, mixture | 1 cup | 292 | 12.4 | 2.4 | n/a | 7.4 | n/a |
| Soup | | | | | | | |
| Hot & sour | 1 cup | 162 | 8.1 | 2.7 | 0.0 | 5.0 | 0.0 |
| Wonton | 1 cup | 52 | 3.0 | 1.0 | 0.0 | 4.0 | 0.0 |
| Spareribs | 4 oz. | 450 | 34.4 | 12.6 | 0.0 | 0.0 | 0.0 |
| Spring roll, vegetable | 1 piece | 158 | 6.9 | 0.9 | 0.0 | 19.9 | 0.4 |
| Vegetables | | | | | | | |
| ■ Steamed | 1 cup | 88 | 0.5 | 0.1 | 0.0 | 18.9 | 5.0 |
| Stir fried | 1 | 86 | 3.0 | 0.5 | 0.0 | 11.0 | 7.0 |
| Wonton, meat, fried | 1 each | 55 | 2.5 | 0.8 | n/a | 4.8 | n/a |
| **Coffee Shop** | | | | | | | |
| Asian chicken salad, no dressing | 1 | 300 | 9.0 | 1.5 | 0.0 | 21.0 | 13.0 |
| Chicken-fried steak & eggs | 1 serv. | 723 | 56.0 | 18.0 | n/a | 31.0 | 2.0 |
| Eggs Benedict | 1 serv. | 860 | 56.0 | 23.0 | 0.0 | 55.0 | 2.0 |
| ■ Egg substitute | 2 oz. | 62 | 1.1 | 0.0 | 0.0 | 4.1 | 0.0 |
| French toast, w/butter | 1 | 178 | 9.4 | 3.9 | n/a | 18.0 | n/a |
| ■ Grits | 4 oz. | 77 | 0.2 | 0.0 | 0.0 | 17.1 | 0.1 |
| Hot fudge sundae | 2 scoops | 569 | 17.3 | 10.1 | 0.0 | 95.3 | n/a |
| ■ Oatmeal | 4 oz. | 69 | 0.5 | 0.1 | 0.0 | 15.3 | 0.0 |

■ Contains less than 20% fat
n/a Not available

25

* See note, page xli

| Item | SERVING | CAL-ORIES | FAT GRAMS | SAT. FAT GRAMS | TRANS FAT GRAMS | CARB. GRAMS | SUGAR GRAMS |
|---|---|---|---|---|---|---|---|
| Omelet, w/cheese & vegetables | 1 | 714 | 53.0 | 10.0 | n/a | 29.0 | 5.0 |
| w/ham & cheddar | 1 | 743 | 55.0 | 10.0 | n/a | 24.0 | 2.0 |
| Sandwiches | | | | | | | |
| Bacon, lettuce & tomato | 1 | 634 | 46.0 | 8.0 | 0.0 | 37.0 | 4.0 |
| Chicken salad | 1 | 460 | 12.0 | 1.5 | 0.0 | 67.0 | 11.0 |
| Club | 1 | 718 | 38.0 | 7.0 | 0.0 | 62.0 | 6.0 |
| Egg salad | 1 | 379 | 26.0 | 4.3 | n/a | 27.3 | 2.9 |
| French dip | 1 | 410 | 16.0 | 9.0 | n/a | 43.0 | n/a |
| Grilled cheese | 1 | 399 | 23.2 | 11.9 | n/a | 30.0 | 3.3 |
| Grilled chicken | 1 | 509 | 19.0 | 5.0 | n/a | 52.0 | 10.0 |
| Ham & swiss, on rye | 1 | 533 | 31.0 | 4.0 | n/a | 40.0 | 9.0 |
| Patty melt | 1 | 695 | 44.0 | 13.0 | n/a | 39.0 | 1.0 |
| Tuna melt | 1 | 641 | 23.0 | 8.0 | n/a | 75.0 | 2.0 |
| Tuna salad | 1 | 326 | 14.4 | 1.9 | n/a | 35.2 | 4.9 |
| Turkey salad club | 1 | 350 | 21.0 | 10.0 | n/a | 9.0 | n/a |
| **Delicatessen** | | | | | | | |
| ■ Applesauce | ½ cup | 97 | 0.2 | 0.0 | 0.0 | 25.4 | n/a |
| ■ Bagel, 3" plain | 1 each | 157 | 0.9 | 0.1 | 0.0 | 30.4 | 0.6 |
| ■ Bialy | 1 | 190 | 2.3 | 0.3 | 0.0 | 36.4 | n/a |
| Blintz, cheese | 1 | 160 | 9.0 | 4.0 | 0.0 | 15.0 | 4.0 |
| ■ Topping, cherry | 2 oz. | 57 | 0.0 | 0.0 | 0.0 | 13.9 | 6.0 |
| Sour cream | 2 tb. | 60 | 5.0 | 3.5 | n/a | 1.0 | 1.0 |
| Bread | | | | | | | |
| Challah | 1 slice | 200 | 7.0 | 1.5 | 0.0 | 29.0 | 4.0 |
| ■ Pumpernickel, dark | 1 slice | 80 | 1.0 | 0.5 | 0.0 | 15.0 | 1.0 |
| ■ Rye, Jewish | 1 slice | 80 | 1.0 | 0.0 | 0.0 | 14.0 | 1.0 |
| Chicken stew, w/potatoes, vegetables, & gravy | 1 cup | 291 | 14.3 | 4.0 | n/a | 15.1 | n/a |
| Chicken liver | 2 oz. | 95 | 3.7 | 1.2 | 0.1 | 0.5 | 0.0 |
| Coleslaw | 6 oz. | 150 | 8.0 | n/a | n/a | 18.0 | n/a |
| Cream cheese, whipped | 1 tsp. | 12 | 1.2 | 0.8 | 0.0 | 0.2 | 0.2 |
| Danish, apple cinnamon | 1 each | 263 | 13.1 | 3.5 | n/a | 33.9 | 19.6 |
| Cheese | 1 each | 266 | 15.6 | 4.8 | n/a | 26.4 | 6.2 |
| Gefilte fish, Manischewitz, no sugar | 1 each | 50 | 1.5 | 0.5 | 0.0 | 0.3 | 0.0 |
| Herring | | | | | | | |
| Pickled | 3 oz. | 223 | 15.3 | 2.0 | 0.0 | 8.2 | 5.0 |
| W/sour cream | 2 oz. | 150 | 10.0 | n/a | n/a | 0.0 | 0.0 |
| Knish, potato | 1 each | 215 | 12.5 | 2.6 | n/a | 20.8 | n/a |
| Knockwurst | 4 oz. | 348 | 31.4 | 11.6 | n/a | 3.6 | 0.0 |
| Kugel, noodle | 1 serv. | 300 | 20.0 | n/a | 0.0 | 26.0 | n/a |
| Lox | 3 oz. | 100 | 3.7 | 0.8 | 0.0 | 0.0 | 0.0 |
| ■ Matzo Brei, w/egg whites | 1 serv. | 161 | 1.6 | 0.3 | 0.0 | 22.0 | 1.0 |
| Potato pancake | 2 oz. | 154 | 8.6 | 1.7 | 0.0 | 16.2 | 0.0 |
| ■ Rice pudding w/raisins | 2 oz. | 165 | 1.0 | 0.0 | 0.0 | 37.0 | 15.0 |
| Rugelach | 1 piece | 115 | 7.0 | 2.0 | n/a | 13.0 | n/a |

■ Contains less than 20% fat
n/a Not available

| Item | SERVING | CAL-ORIES | FAT GRAMS | SAT. FAT GRAMS | TRANS FAT GRAMS | CARB. GRAMS | SUGAR GRAMS |
|---|---|---|---|---|---|---|---|
| **Salad** | | | | | | | |
| Macaroni | ½ cup | 197 | 9.1 | 1.5 | 0.0 | 25.0 | 7.6 |
| Potato | ½ cup | 163 | 8.6 | 1.5 | 0.0 | 19.3 | n/a |
| **Sandwiches** | | | | | | | |
| Corned beef & Swiss, w/rye | 1 each | 427 | 25.7 | 9.5 | n/a | 21.7 | 5.3 |
| Pastrami | 1 each | 331 | 18.1 | 6.2 | n/a | 27.3 | n/a |
| Salami | 1 each | 234 | 11.1 | 3.4 | n/a | 24.8 | n/a |
| Turkey | 1 each | 346 | 14.2 | 1.9 | n/a | 29.5 | 2.3 |
| Short ribs, beef, boiled | 4 oz. | 328 | 20.9 | 8.3 | n/a | 0.0 | 0.0 |
| **Soup** | | | | | | | |
| Borscht/beet | 1 cup | 78 | 4.0 | 2.4 | n/a | 8.3 | n/a |
| Chicken, w/matzo balls | ½ cup | 80 | 4.0 | 2.0 | 0.0 | 9.0 | 0.0 |
| Chicken w/rice | 1 cup | 60 | 1.9 | 0.5 | 0.0 | 7.2 | 0.2 |
| Mushroom barley | 1 cup | 73 | 2.3 | 0.4 | 0.0 | 11.7 | 0.0 |
| * Split pea, vegetarian | 1 cup | 190 | 4.4 | 1.8 | 0.0 | 28.0 | 0.0 |
| *■ Sweet & sour cabbage | 1 cup | 60 | 0.0 | 0.0 | 0.0 | n/a | n/a |
| | | | | | | | |
| **French** | | | | | | | |
| Bananas flambé | 1 banana | 465 | 20.0 | n/a | n/a | n/a | n/a |
| Beef Provençal | 4 oz. beef | 265 | 15.0 | n/a | n/a | n/a | n/a |
| Boulllabaisse (made w/fish fillets, shrimp, crab or lobster, & clams or oysters) | 1 cup | 241 | 8.9 | 2.0 | 0.0 | 4.8 | 0.0 |
| Caviar | 3 oz. | 214 | 15.2 | 3.5 | 0.0 | 3.4 | 0.0 |
| ■ Cherries jubilee | ½ cup | 161 | 0.0 | 0.0 | 0.0 | 40.2 | 26.1 |
| ■ Chicken, breast, poached, w/tomato coulis | 1 each | 161 | 3.3 | n/a | n/a | n/a | n/a |
| Chicken Cordon Bleu | 1 each | 494 | 29.0 | 15.4 | n/a | 11.0 | n/a |
| Coquilles St. Jacques | 6 | 300 | 14.0 | n/a | n/a | 2.0 | n/a |
| ■ Crepe, plain | 1.5 oz. | 100 | 1.7 | 0.0 | 0.0 | 16.6 | 6.6 |
| meat filled | 1 each | 194 | 11.3 | 6.0 | n/a | 8.5 | 1.3 |
| Suzette | 1 each | 159 | 9.0 | 3.8 | n/a | 15.6 | n/a |
| Duck à l'Orange | 1 serv. | 780 | 35.0 | n/a | n/a | 47.0 | n/a |
| ■ Escargot | 4 each | 55 | 0.2 | 0.0 | 0.0 | 3.1 | 1.6 |
| Lamb, rack, lean | 3 oz. | 200 | 11.0 | 3.9 | n/a | 0.0 | 0.0 |
| Lemon meringue | 1 each | 301 | 13.6 | 2.9 | n/a | 41.1 | n/a |
| Chocolate mousse | ½ cup | 105 | 5.0 | 4.0 | n/a | 13.0 | 8.0 |
| Onion soup, au gratin | 1 cup | 284 | 15.6 | n/a | n/a | n/a | n/a |
| Pate de foie gras | 2 oz. | 262 | 24.9 | 8.2 | n/a | 2.7 | n/a |
| Quiche Lorraine | 6 oz. | 509 | 39.5 | 18.2 | n/a | 24.2 | n/a |
| *■ Ratatouille | 1 cup | 105 | 1.0 | 0.0 | 0.0 | 21.0 | 7.0 |
| Soufflé, cheese | 1 serv. | 192 | 13.9 | 5.1 | n/a | 5.7 | 3.2 |
| Truffle, chocolate | 1 | 78 | 6.0 | 4.0 | n/a | 5.0 | 5.0 |

■ Contains less than 20% fat
n/a Not available

* See note, page xli

| Item | SERVING | CAL-ORIES | FAT GRAMS | SAT. FAT GRAMS | TRANS FAT GRAMS | CARB. GRAMS | SUGAR GRAMS |
|---|---|---|---|---|---|---|---|
| **Indian** | | | | | | | |
| Bread | | | | | | | |
| ■ Chapatti | 1 each | 120 | 2.5 | 0.0 | 0.0 | 20.0 | 1.0 |
| ■ Naan, Tandoori style | 1 serv. | 200 | 4.0 | 1.0 | 0.0 | 35.0 | 2.0 |
| * ■ Dal Bahaar | 3.5 oz. | 300 | 6.0 | 0.5 | n/a | 53.0 | 0.0 |
| Ghee | 1 tb. | 112 | 12.7 | 7.9 | n/a | 0.0 | 0.0 |
| Lamb curry, biryani | 6 oz. | 424 | 23.3 | n/a | n/a | 42.2 | n/a |
| ■ Lassi, mango | 1 serv. | 210 | 1.5 | n/a | n/a | 48.0 | n/a |
| Paratha | 2.8 oz. | 290 | 9.0 | n/a | n/a | 42.0 | n/a |
| * Raita | ½ cup | 125 | 7.0 | n/a | 0.0 | 12.0 | n/a |
| Spinach dal and basmati rice | 1 serv. | 377 | 9.0 | 1.0 | 0.0 | 62.0 | 4.0 |
| Tandoori chicken w/spinach | 1 serv. | 330 | 10.0 | 2.0 | 0.0 | 39.0 | 3.0 |
| Vegetable curry | 3.5 oz. | 83 | 2.4 | n/a | 0.0 | 12.3 | n/a |
| | | | | | | | |
| **Italian** | | | | | | | |
| Biscuit, tortoni | 1 | 235 | 23.0 | n/a | n/a | n/a | n/a |
| Bread | | | | | | | |
| Garlic | 1 piece | 160 | 10.0 | 3.0 | n/a | 14.0 | 2.0 |
| ■ Italian | 1 piece | 54 | 0.7 | 0.2 | 0.0 | 10.0 | 0.2 |
| Stick, sesame | 3 each | 44 | 1.5 | 0.3 | 0.0 | 6.6 | 0.4 |
| Calamari, fried | 3 oz. | 149 | 6.4 | 1.6 | 0.0 | 6.6 | n/a |
| ■ Cappuccino, w/nonfat milk | 6 oz. | 56 | 0.0 | 0.0 | 0.0 | 7.6 | 6.9 |
| Cappuccino, w/whole milk | 6 oz. | 98 | 4.9 | 3.1 | n/a | 7.7 | 7.0 |
| Cheese, parmesan, grated | 1 tb. | 22 | 1.4 | 0.9 | n/a | 0.2 | 0.0 |
| Fettuccine alfredo | 10 oz. | 368 | 16.8 | 7.4 | n/a | 42.1 | 5.3 |
| Gnocchi | | | | | | | |
| Cheese | 1 cup | 128 | 8.5 | 3.3 | n/a | 6.0 | n/a |
| Potato | 1 cup | 268 | 13.1 | 8.0 | n/a | 33.1 | n/a |
| ■ Ice, Italian | ½ cup | 61 | 0.0 | 0.0 | 0.0 | 15.7 | n/a |
| Linguini, w/red clam sauce | 1 each | 290 | 8.0 | 2.5 | 0.0 | 44.0 | 5.0 |
| w/white sauce | 1 cup | 378 | 10.0 | 5.0 | 0.0 | 56.0 | 3.0 |
| ■ Mussels, marinara | 1 cup | 269 | 5.6 | 1.1 | 0.0 | 23.7 | n/a |
| Pasta | | | | | | | |
| Al pesto | 1 cup | 330 | 10.0 | 4.8 | 0.0 | 51.0 | 6.0 |
| Carbonara | 1 cup | 284 | 8.0 | 4.0 | 0.0 | 43.0 | 3.0 |
| ■ Spaghetti, w/marinara sauce | 1 serv. | 490 | 8.0 | 1.5 | 0.0 | 90.0 | 17.0 |
| Primavera | 1 cup | 330 | 16.0 | 4.0 | 0.0 | 39.0 | 6.0 |
| w/tomato and basil | 1 cup | 330 | 10.4 | 4.8 | 0.0 | 51.0 | 6.0 |
| ■ Polenta | 1 cup | 85 | 0.8 | 0.0 | 0.0 | 16.0 | 2.0 |
| ■ Ravioli, spinach w/tomato sauce | 1 serv. | 370 | 3.0 | 1.1 | 0.0 | 53.0 | 2.0 |
| ■ Risotto, wild mushroom | 1 serv | 217 | 1.0 | 0.5 | 0.0 | 47.0 | 1.0 |
| Salad | | | | | | | |
| Antipasto, w/peppered salami | 1 cup | 134 | 10.0 | 3.0 | n/a | 6.0 | 2.0 |
| Tomato & mozzarella | 1 cup | 360 | 28.0 | n/a | n/a | 20.0 | 0.0 |
| ■ Tomato and onion | 1 serv. | 44 | 0.0 | 0.0 | 0.0 | 10.0 | n/a |
| Shrimp scampi | 1 serv. | 311 | 22.2 | 12.9 | 0.0 | 1.2 | n/a |

■ Contains less than 20% fat
n/a Not available

* See note, page xli

| Item | SERVING | CAL-ORIES | FAT GRAMS | SAT. FAT GRAMS | TRANS FAT GRAMS | CARB. GRAMS | SUGAR GRAMS |
|---|---|---|---|---|---|---|---|
| **Soup** | | | | | | | |
| Minestrone | 1 cup | 82 | 2.5 | 0.6 | 0.0 | 11.2 | 0.0 |
| ■ Tortellini, w/chicken & vegetables | 1 cup | 110 | 2.0 | 1.0 | 0.0 | 18.0 | 4.0 |
| Tiramisu | 1 serv. | 240 | 29.0 | n/a | n/a | 30.0 | 29.0 |
| **Veal** | | | | | | | |
| Parmigiana | 4 oz. | 133 | 6.9 | 2.1 | n/a | 13.7 | 3.7 |
| Scaloppine | 1 serv. | 238 | 16.9 | 4.8 | n/a | 1.4 | n/a |
| ■ Osso buco w/risotto | 1 serv. | 490 | 10.0 | n/a | n/a | n/a | n/a |
| **Vegetables** | | | | | | | |
| Broccoli, sautéed w/garlic and oil | ½ cup | 75 | 5.0 | 0.5 | 0.0 | 5.0 | 1.0 |
| Broccoli raab | 3 oz. | 28 | 0.4 | 0.1 | 0.0 | 2.7 | 0.5 |
| Escarole, braised | ½ cup | 60 | 4.0 | n/a | 0.0 | n/a | n/a |
| ■ Peppers, roasted | ½ cup | 30 | 0.0 | 0.0 | 0.0 | 5.0 | 4.0 |
| Zabaglione | 1 serv. | 77 | 3.5 | n/a | n/a | n/a | n/a |
| **Japanese** | | | | | | | |
| Beef, w/teriyaki sauce | 4 oz. | 257 | 13.7 | 5.1 | n/a | 9.1 | n/a |
| Chicken | 1 each | 510 | 13.0 | 2.5 | n/a | 71.0 | 22.0 |
| ■ Noodles, soba | ½ cup | 56 | 0.1 | 0.0 | 0.0 | 12.2 | 0.0 |
| ■ Udon | ½ cup | 57 | 0.3 | n/a | 0.0 | 11.5 | n/a |
| **Sushi** | | | | | | | |
| ■ California roll, real crab | 3 pieces | 107 | 1.0 | 0.0 | 0.0 | 26.7 | 2.0 |
| ■ Cucumber roll | 3 pieces | 60 | 0.5 | 0.0 | 0.0 | 12.5 | 1.0 |
| ■ Tuna roll | 3 pieces | 75 | 0.0 | 0.0 | 0.0 | 15.0 | 1.0 |
| ■ Spicy | 3 pieces | 93 | 0.3 | 0.0 | 0.0 | 17.2 | 1.3 |
| ■ Vegetarian roll | 3 pieces | 93 | 1.3 | 0.0 | 0.0 | 18.0 | 2.0 |
| Sashimi, mackerel | 1 serv. | 45 | 2.2 | 0.6 | 0.0 | 0.0 | 0.0 |
| Tuna | 1 each | 408 | 4.0 | 1.3 | 0.0 | 0.0 | 0.0 |
| Vegetables, tempura | 3 oz. | 138 | 8.6 | 1.7 | n/a | 12.1 | 1.5 |
| **Mexican** | | | | | | | |
| Arroz con pollo | 1 serv. | 500 | 23 | n/a | n/a | 50.0 | n/a |
| ■ Beans, refried | ½ cup | 150 | 3.0 | 1.0 | n/a | 24.0 | 0.0 |
| fat free | ½ cup | 100 | 0.0 | 0.0 | 0.0 | 18.0 | 1.0 |
| Burrito, bean | 1 each | 224 | 6.8 | 3.4 | n/a | 35.7 | n/a |
| Beef | 1 each | 415 | 18.9 | 6.4 | n/a | 39.4 | n/a |
| Chicken breast w/mole | 1 each | 250 | 10.0 | n/a | n/a | n/a | n/a |
| Chili rellenos | 1 serv. | 524 | 40.0 | 23.0 | n/a | 9.0 | 6.0 |
| Chimichanga, beef | 1 each | 425 | 19.7 | 8.5 | n/a | 42.8 | n/a |
| Empanada, turkey or chicken | 1 each | 550 | 30.0 | n/a | n/a | n/a | n/a |
| Enchilada, beef & cheese | 1 each | 323 | 17.6 | 9.1 | n/a | 30.5 | n/a |
| Enchilada, chicken | 1 each | 283 | 9.7 | 3.7 | n/a | 33.2 | n/a |
| Fajitas, beef | 1 each | 399 | 18.2 | 5.5 | n/a | 35.7 | n/a |
| Chicken | 1 each | 363 | 12.0 | 2.3 | n/a | 44.3 | n/a |
| ■ Flan | ½ cup | 140 | 2.5 | 1.5 | n/a | 26.0 | 25.0 |

■ Contains less than 20% fat
n/a Not available

| Item | SERVING | CAL-ORIES | FAT GRAMS | SAT. FAT GRAMS | TRANS FAT GRAMS | CARB. GRAMS | SUGAR GRAMS |
|---|---|---|---|---|---|---|---|
| Guacamole | ⅓ cup | 77 | 5.3 | 0.0 | 0.0 | 5.3 | n/a |
| Huevos rancheros | 1 each | 465 | 15.0 | n/a | n/a | n/a | n/a |
| Menudo | 1 each | 278 | 8.2 | n/a | n/a | n/a | n/a |
| Nachos, w/cheese | 1 serv. | 323 | 19.0 | 4.5 | n/a | 33.0 | 3.0 |
| Quesadilla | 1 each | 183 | 9.5 | 3.5 | n/a | 18.3 | n/a |
| ■ Salsa | 1 tb. | 4 | 0.0 | 0.0 | 0.0 | 1.0 | 0.5 |
| ■ Sangria | 6 fl.oz. | 118 | 0.0 | 0.0 | 0.0 | 15.8 | n/a |
| Soup | | | | | | | |
| ■   Black bean | 1 cup | 116 | 1.5 | 0.4 | 0.0 | 19.8 | 0.2 |
| ■   Gazpacho | 1 cup | 46 | 0.2 | 0.0 | 0.0 | 4.4 | 2.2 |
| Taco, beef | 1 each | 291 | 18.0 | 6.0 | n/a | 21.0 | 1.0 |
| Taco, fish | 1 each | 290 | 16.0 | 3.0 | 0.0 | 30.0 | 2.0 |
| Tortilla chips | 1 oz. | 150 | 8.0 | 1.0 | 0.0 | 18.0 | 1.0 |
| Tortilla, flour, 6" | 1 each | 90 | 3.0 | 0.0 | 0.0 | 13.0 | 0.0 |
| ■   corn, 6" | 1 each | 70 | 1.0 | 0.0 | 0.0 | 14.0 | 0.0 |
| Tostados, beef, w/guacamole and salsa | 1 each | 300 | 14.0 | 5.0 | n/a | n/a | n/a |
| **Middle Eastern/Greek** | | | | | | | |
| Baba ghanoush | 2 tb. | 140 | 6.0 | 0.0 | 0.0 | 16.0 | 0.0 |
| ■ Bread, pita, 6½" | 1 each | 165 | 0.7 | 0.1 | 0.0 | 33.4 | 0.8 |
| ■ Couscous, cooked | ½ cup | 88 | 0.1 | 0.0 | 0.0 | 18.2 | 0.1 |
| Falafel, patty, 2¼" | 1 each | 57 | 3.0 | 0.4 | n/a | 5.4 | n/a |
| Hummus | 2 tb. | 46 | 2.7 | 0.4 | 0.0 | 4.0 | n/a |
| Kabob, shish | 2.5 oz. | 130 | 7.0 | n/a | n/a | 2.0 | n/a |
| Lamb | 4 oz. | 211 | 8.3 | 3.0 | n/a | 0.0 | 0.0 |
| Kibbeh | 1 cup | 450 | 18.0 | n/a | n/a | 28.0 | n/a |
| Moussaka, lamb & eggplant | 1 serv. | 238 | 13.0 | 4.6 | 0.0 | 13.1 | 6.9 |
| Salad, classic Greek | 1 cup | 50 | 4.0 | 0.8 | 0.0 | 2.5 | 1.5 |
| ■ Soup, lentil | 1 cup | 140 | 0.0 | 0.0 | 0.0 | 24.0 | 5.0 |
| Spanakopita | 1 each | 60 | 2.0 | 1.0 | 0.0 | 8.0 | 0.0 |
| Tabouli/tabbouleh | ¼ cup | 50 | 3.8 | 0.5 | 0.0 | 4.0 | 0.0 |
| **Seafood** | | | | | | | |
| Butter, melted | 1 tb. | 110 | 12.5 | 7.8 | 0.0 | 0.0 | 0.0 |
| Chowder | | | | | | | |
| *   Clam, Manhattan | 8 oz. | 127 | 3.2 | 2.0 | 0.0 | 17.8 | 3.8 |
|     New England | 6 oz. | 153 | 8.9 | 3.8 | n/a | 13.4 | 0.6 |
| ■     Reduced fat | 6 oz. | 70 | 1.0 | 0.3 | n/a | 12.1 | 1.3 |
|   Fish | 8 oz. | 180 | 5.0 | 2.2 | 0.0 | 11.0 | 3.3 |
| Clams | | | | | | | |
| Fried | 4 oz. | 373 | 19.3 | n/a | n/a | 38.7 | 4.0 |
| ■   Raw | 6 each | 64 | 0.8 | 0.1 | 0.0 | 2.2 | 0.0 |
| ■   Steamers | 12 each | 180 | 1.0 | n/a | 0.0 | n/a | 0.0 |
| Crab, deviled | 1 serv. | 346 | 17.8 | 3.6 | n/a | 23.5 | n/a |
| Crab cakes | 2 oz. | 88 | 4.3 | 0.8 | n/a | 0.3 | n/a |
| Fish & chips | 1 each | 780 | 39.0 | 9.0 | n/a | 86.0 | 2.0 |

■ Contains less than 20% fat
n/a Not available

* See note, page xli

| Item | SERVING | CAL-ORIES | FAT GRAMS | SAT. FAT GRAMS | TRANS FAT GRAMS | CARB. GRAMS | SUGAR GRAMS |
|---|---|---|---|---|---|---|---|
| ■ Flounder, fillet, baked/broiled | 3.5 oz. | 116 | 1.5 | 0.4 | 0.0 | 0.0 | 0.0 |
| Fried | 4 oz. | 252 | 13.0 | 2.8 | n/a | 9.6 | n/a |
| * ■ Halibut, baked/broiled | 6 oz. | 238 | 5.0 | 0.7 | 0.0 | 0.0 | 0.0 |
| Lobster | | | | | | | |
| Baked/broiled | 8 oz. | 265 | 6.9 | 3.7 | 0.0 | 2.8 | 0.0 |
| Newberg | 1 serv. | 551 | 44.9 | 26.7 | n/a | 10.2 | 5.3 |
| ■ Steamed, whole | 1.5 lb. | 172 | 1.0 | 0.2 | n/a | 2.2 | 0.0 |
| Thermidor | 1 serv. | 852 | 69.4 | 41.3 | n/a | 15.8 | 8.2 |
| Oysters, fried | 4 oz. | 301 | 14.6 | 3.7 | n/a | 32.5 | n/a |
| Raw | 6 each | 243 | 6.9 | 1.5 | n/a | 14.9 | n/a |
| Stew | 8 fl.oz. | 135 | 7.9 | 5.1 | n/a | 9.8 | n/a |
| Salmon, steamed/poached, wild | 3.5 oz. | 183 | 7.4 | 1.6 | 0.0 | 0.0 | 0.0 |
| ■ Sauce, cocktail | 1 tb. | 25 | 0.0 | 0.0 | 0.0 | 6.0 | 5.5 |
| Tartar | 1 tb. | 45 | 4.5 | 0.8 | n/a | 2.0 | 1.0 |
| Low cal | 1 tb. | 31 | 2.5 | 0.4 | n/a | 2.3 | n/a |
| Shrimp, battered/fried | 3.5 oz. | 314 | 21.0 | 7.0 | n/a | 21.0 | 0.0 |
| ■ Boiled | 3.5 oz. | 98 | 1.1 | 0.3 | 0.0 | 0.0 | 0.0 |
| Trout, rainbow, cooked | 6 oz. | 283 | 12.2 | 4.1 | 0.0 | 0.0 | 0.0 |
| **Steak House** | | | | | | | |
| ■ BBQ chicken breast | 10 oz. | 280 | 5.0 | 2.0 | n/a | n/a | n/a |
| Beef, untrimmed | 12 oz. | 791 | 58.9 | 23.1 | n/a | 0.0 | 0.0 |
| Buffalo wings | 6 pieces | 295 | 20.9 | 5.4 | n/a | 0.2 | 0.1 |
| Caesar salad | 2 cups | 311 | 25.4 | 4.1 | n/a | 14.8 | 4.9 |
| Cheese fries | 2 cups | 1190 | 75.5 | 39.5 | n/a | n/a | n/a |
| Filet mignon, trimmed of fat | 9 oz. | 579 | 41.8 | 16.7 | n/a | 0.0 | 0.0 |
| Untrimmed | 9 oz. | 592 | 43.6 | 17.9 | n/a | 0.0 | 0.0 |
| House salad, w/fat-free dressing | 1 serv. | 170 | 4.0 | 0.0 | 0.0 | n/a | n/a |
| New York steak, trimmed | 12 oz. | 570 | 34.0 | 18.0 | n/a | 0.0 | 0.0 |
| Pork chop | 12 oz. | 630 | 36.1 | 13.6 | n/a | 0.0 | 0.0 |
| Porterhouse steak, untrimmed | 12 oz. | 851 | 66.8 | 26.3 | n/a | 0.0 | 0.0 |
| Potato skins w/bacon & cheese | 1 each | 70 | 4.0 | 1.3 | n/a | 6.4 | 0.3 |
| Prime rib, trimmed | 12 oz. | 915 | 72.0 | 29.8 | n/a | 0.0 | 0.0 |
| untrimmed | 12 oz. | 941 | 75.3 | 31.9 | n/a | 0.0 | 0.0 |
| Rib eye, trimmed | 12 oz. | 644 | 40.7 | 15.8 | n/a | 0.0 | 0.0 |
| Sirloin, trimmed | 12 oz. | 768 | 56.7 | 22.8 | n/a | 0.0 | 0.0 |
| untrimmed | 12 oz. | 806 | 61.6 | 25.5 | n/a | 0.0 | 0.0 |
| T-bone steak, trimmed | 12 oz. | 724 | 50.3 | 19.6 | n/a | 0.0 | 0.0 |
| **Thai** | | | | | | | |
| ■ Basil chicken | 1 serv. | 427 | 13.5 | 2.7 | n/a | 17.8 | 9.8 |
| ■ Beef peanut satay, Thai style | 1 serv. | 286 | 18.1 | 5.9 | n/a | 4.9 | 1.7 |
| ■ Fried rice, Thai style | 1 each | 402 | 13.6 | 2.0 | n/a | 62.2 | 2.6 |
| Noodles mee krob | | | | | | | |
| Crunchy, w/chicken, pork & shrimp | 1 serv. | 550 | 15.0 | n/a | n/a | n/a | n/a |

■ Contains less than 20% fat
n/a Not available

31

\* See note, page xli

| Item | SERVING | CAL-ORIES | FAT GRAMS | SAT. FAT GRAMS | TRANS FAT GRAMS | CARB. GRAMS | SUGAR GRAMS |
|---|---|---|---|---|---|---|---|
| Soft fried, w/pork, shrimp & vegetables | 1 serv. | 560 | 30.0 | n/a | n/a | n/a | n/a |
| ■ Pad Thai, w/shrimp | 1 serv. | 293 | 10.1 | 1.6 | n/a | 36.1 | 10.9 |
| ■ Vegetarian | 1 serv. | 407 | 22.5 | 4.3 | n/a | 39.8 | 11.3 |
| ■ Peanut chicken w/rice, Thai style | 1 serv. | 272 | 10.5 | 2.3 | n/a | 25.8 | 3.3 |
| Red curry chicken, Thai style | 1 serv. | 367 | 26.5 | 19.5 | n/a | 9.2 | 3.4 |
| ■ Salad, chicken, broiled, Thai style | 1 serv. | 257 | 7.2 | 1.9 | n/a | 24.5 | 4.4 |
| Soup | | | | | | | |
| ■ Spicy Thai | 1 each | 240 | 2.0 | 0.0 | 0.0 | 48.0 | 6.0 |
| ■ Hot & sour, Thai | 1 each | 111 | 1.5 | 0.3 | 0.0 | 10.3 | 2.0 |
| ■ Spicy noodles, Thai style | 1 serv. | 626 | 26.1 | 4.4 | n/a | 64.7 | 7.3 |
| ■ Spicy vegetables, lemongrass Thai | 1 serv. | 239 | 16.3 | 2.6 | n/a | 19.4 | 4.9 |
| ■ Spring roll, vegetable, Thai style | 1 piece | 158 | 6.9 | 0.9 | 0.0 | 19.9 | 4.6 |
| ■ Tofu w/sour curry, Thai style | 1 serv. | 424 | 31.9 | 4.3 | n/a | 15.9 | 3.5 |

## EGGS, EGG DISHES, & EGG SUBSTITUTES

### Eggs
Chicken

| Item | SERVING | CAL-ORIES | FAT GRAMS | SAT. FAT GRAMS | TRANS FAT GRAMS | CARB. GRAMS | SUGAR GRAMS |
|---|---|---|---|---|---|---|---|
| Fried in butter | 1 | 92 | 7.0 | 2.0 | n/a | 0.4 | 0.4 |
| Hard or soft boiled | 1 | 78 | 5.3 | 1.6 | 0.0 | 0.6 | 0.6 |
| Poached | 1 | 74 | 5.0 | 1.5 | 0.0 | 0.4 | 0.4 |
| Scrambled w/milk and butter | 1 | 101 | 7.5 | 2.2 | n/a | 1.3 | 1.1 |
| ■ White | 1 | 17 | 0.1 | 0.0 | 0.0 | 0.2 | 0.2 |
| Yolk | 1 | 53 | 4.4 | 1.6 | 0.0 | 0.6 | 0.1 |
| Duck | 1 | 130 | 9.6 | 2.6 | 0.0 | 1.0 | 0.7 |
| Goose | 1 | 266 | 19.1 | 5.2 | 0.0 | 1.9 | 1.4 |
| Quail | 1 | 14 | 1.0 | 0.3 | 0.0 | 0.0 | 0.0 |

### Egg Dishes

| Item | SERVING | CAL-ORIES | FAT GRAMS | SAT. FAT GRAMS | TRANS FAT GRAMS | CARB. GRAMS | SUGAR GRAMS |
|---|---|---|---|---|---|---|---|
| * ■ Frittata, no cholesterol | 1 serv. | 92 | 0.4 | 0.0 | 0.0 | n/a | n/a |
| Omelet, veggie-cheese | 1 serv. | 480 | 39.0 | 13.0 | n/a | 9.0 | 4.0 |
| ■ Omelet, only whites w/veggies and cheese | 1 serv. | 175 | 2.0 | n/a | 0.0 | 22.0 | n/a |
| Quiche, bacon & cheese | 6 oz. | 520 | 37.0 | 18.0 | n/a | 30.0 | n/a |
| Quiche, cheese, no meat | 6 oz. | 504 | 39.1 | 19.0 | n/a | 23.7 | n/a |
| Quiche, spinach, vegetarian | 6 oz. | 408 | 31.1 | 14.4 | n/a | 19.6 | n/a |

### Egg Substitutes

| Item | SERVING | CAL-ORIES | FAT GRAMS | SAT. FAT GRAMS | TRANS FAT GRAMS | CARB. GRAMS | SUGAR GRAMS |
|---|---|---|---|---|---|---|---|
| ■ Better 'N Eggs | ¼ cup | 25 | 0.0 | 0.0 | 0.0 | 0.5 | 0.5 |
| ■ Egg Beaters | ¼ cup | 30 | 0.0 | 0.0 | 0.0 | 1.0 | 1.0 |
| ■ Egg Replacer, Ener-G Foods | 1.5 tsp. | 14 | 0.0 | 0.0 | 0.0 | 3.7 | 0.0 |
| ■ Egg whites, dried | 2 tsp. | 17 | 0.0 | 0.0 | 0.0 | 0.4 | 0.2 |
| ■ Scramblers, Morningstar Farms | ¼ cup | 39 | 0.4 | n/a | 0.0 | 2.3 | 1.4 |
| ■ Second Nature | ¼ cup | 30 | 0.0 | 0.0 | 0.0 | n/a | n/a |
| ■ Tofutti Egg Watchers | ¼ cup | 30 | 0.0 | 0.0 | 0.0 | 1.0 | 1.0 |

■ Contains less than 20% fat
n/a Not available

32

* See note, page xli

| Item | SERVING | CAL-ORIES | FAT GRAMS | SAT. FAT GRAMS | TRANS FAT GRAMS | CARB. GRAMS | SUGAR GRAMS |
|---|---|---|---|---|---|---|---|

## FAST FOOD

Restaurants and fast food and takeout establishments are **not required** to provide a nutritional analysis.

| Item | SERVING | CAL-ORIES | FAT GRAMS | SAT. FAT GRAMS | TRANS FAT GRAMS | CARB. GRAMS | SUGAR GRAMS |
|---|---|---|---|---|---|---|---|
| **Arby's** | | | | | | | |
| Beef 'n Cheddar Sandwich | 1 | 440 | 21.0 | 7.0 | 2.0 | 44.0 | 8.0 |
| Chicken, Bacon 'n Swiss | 1 | 550 | 27.0 | 7.0 | 0.0 | 49.0 | 10.0 |
| Breast Fillet, crispy | 1 | 500 | 25.0 | 4.0 | 1.0 | 48.0 | 8.0 |
| Southwest Chicken Wrap | 1 | 550 | 30.0 | 11.0 | 1.0 | 45.0 | 1.0 |
| Cookie, Chocolate Gourmet | 1 | 200 | 10.0 | 6.0 | 2.0 | 26.0 | 16.0 |
| Curly fries, large | 1 serv. | 630 | 34.0 | 5.0 | 7.0 | 73.0 | n/a |
| Small | 1 serv. | 340 | 18.0 | 3.0 | 3.0 | 39.0 | n/a |
| Milk shake, chocolate, regular | 1 | 510 | 13.0 | 8.0 | 0.0 | 83.0 | 81.0 |
| Roast Beef Sandwich, regular | 1 | 320 | 13.0 | 6.0 | 1.0 | 34.0 | 5.0 |
| Giant | 1 | 450 | 19.0 | 9.0 | 2.0 | 41.0 | 6.0 |
| Junior | 1 | 270 | 9.0 | 4.0 | 0.5 | 34.0 | 5.0 |
| Super | 1 | 440 | 19.0 | 7.0 | 1.0 | 48.0 | 11.0 |
| Roast Turkey & Swiss Sandwich | 1 | 720 | 27.0 | 6.0 | 1.0 | 74.0 | 16.0 |
| Salad, Chicken Club | 1 | 530 | 33.0 | 10.0 | 1.0 | 32.0 | 4.0 |
| Martha's Vineyard | 1 | 250 | 8.0 | 4.5 | 0.0 | 23.0 | 23.0 |
| Santa Fe | 1 | 520 | 29.0 | 9.0 | 1.0 | 40.0 | 6.0 |
| Sauces & Dressings | | | | | | | |
| ■ Arby's Sauce | 1 packet | 15 | 0.0 | 0.0 | 0.0 | 4.0 | 1.0 |
| ■ Bronco Berry | 1 serv. | 120 | 0.0 | 0.0 | 0.0 | 30.0 | 28.0 |
| Buttermilk Ranch Dressing | 1 packet | 290 | 30.0 | 5.0 | 1.0 | 3.0 | 2.0 |
| Horsey Sauce | 1 packet | 60 | 5.0 | 1.0 | 0.0 | 3.0 | 1.0 |
| ■ Ketchup | 1 packet | 20 | 0.0 | 0.0 | 0.0 | 4.0 | 3.0 |
| Mayonnaise, packet | 1 packet | 100 | 11.0 | 2.0 | 2.0 | 0.0 | 0.0 |
| Light | 1 packet | 45 | 4.5 | 1.0 | 0.0 | 1.0 | 0.0 |
| Raspberry Vinaigrette | 1 serv. | 190 | 14.0 | 1.5 | 0.0 | 18.0 | 16.0 |
| Red Ranch Sauce | 1 serv. | 70 | 6.0 | 1.0 | 0.0 | 5.0 | 4.0 |
| **Baja Fresh** | | | | | | | |
| ■ Black Beans | 1 serv. | 360 | 2.5 | 1.0 | 0.0 | 61.0 | n/a |
| Burritos | | | | | | | |
| Baja Charbroiled Chicken | 1 | 930 | 45.0 | 16.0 | 1.0 | 83.0 | n/a |
| Charbroiled Steak | 1 | 1030 | 52.0 | 19.0 | 2.0 | 83.0 | n/a |
| Bean & Cheese Burrito, no meat | 1 | 980 | 40.0 | 18.0 | 1.5 | 114.0 | n/a |
| ■ Veggie & Cheese Bare Burrito, no tortilla | 1 | 580 | 10.0 | 4.0 | 0.0 | 101.0 | n/a |
| Kids | | | | | | | |
| Bean & Cheese Burrito, 8" | 1 | 620 | 18.0 | 7.0 | 0.5 | 93.0 | n/a |
| Chicken Taquitos | 2 | 700 | 37.0 | 7.0 | 1.0 | 69.0 | n/a |
| Quesadilla, cheese | 1 | 610 | 26.0 | 13.0 | 1.0 | 72.0 | n/a |

■ Contains less than 20% fat
n/a Not available

| Item | SERVING | CAL-ORIES | FAT GRAMS | SAT. FAT GRAMS | TRANS FAT GRAMS | CARB. GRAMS | SUGAR GRAMS |
|---|---|---|---|---|---|---|---|
| Nachos | | | | | | | |
| Cheese | 1 order | 1890 | 108.0 | 40.0 | 4.0 | 163.0 | n/a |
| Pico de Gallo | 1 cup | 50 | 0.5 | 0.0 | 0.0 | 12.0 | n/a |
| Pronto Guacamole w/chips | 1 serv. | 560 | 34.0 | 3.0 | 1.0 | 60.0 | n/a |
| Quesadillas | | | | | | | |
| Charbroiled Chicken | 1 order | 1330 | 80.0 | 37.0 | 2.5 | 84.0 | n/a |
| Cheese | 1 order | 1200 | 78.0 | 37.0 | 2.5 | 84.0 | n/a |
| ■ Rice | 1 serv. | 280 | 4.0 | 1.5 | 0.0 | 55.0 | n/a |
| Salads & Dressings | | | | | | | |
| Baja Ensalada | | | | | | | |
| Charbroiled Steak | 1 | 450 | 18.0 | 7.0 | 1.0 | 18.0 | n/a |
| Charbroiled Chicken | 1 | 310 | 7.0 | 2.0 | 0.0 | 18.0 | n/a |
| Charbroiled Mahi-Mahi | 1 serv. | 310 | 12.0 | 3.0 | 0.0 | 22.0 | n/a |
| Charbroiled Shrimp | 1 | 230 | 6.0 | 2.0 | 0.0 | 18.0 | n/a |
| Chipotle Glazed Charbroiled Chicken | 1 | 590 | 22.0 | 6.0 | 1.0 | 54.0 | n/a |
| Served w/Chipotle Vinaigrette | 1 serv. | 110 | 9.0 | 1.0 | 0.0 | 8.0 | n/a |
| Tostada, Charbroiled Chicken | 1 | 1140 | 55.0 | 14.0 | 1.0 | 98.0 | n/a |
| Charbroiled Steak | 1 | 1230 | 63.0 | 17.0 | 2.0 | 98.0 | n/a |
| No Meat | 1 | 1010 | 53.0 | 13.0 | 1.0 | 98.0 | n/a |
| Savory Pork Carnitas | 1 | 570 | 40.0 | 13.0 | 0.0 | 16.0 | n/a |
| Salad Dressings, additional | | | | | | | |
| Olive Oil Vinaigrette | 1 serv. | 290 | 31.0 | 4.5 | 0.0 | 2.0 | n/a |
| Ranch Dressing | 1 serv. | 260 | 26.0 | 6.0 | 0.5 | 2.0 | n/a |
| ■ Fat Free Salsa Verde | 1 serv. | 15 | 0.0 | 0.0 | 0.0 | 3.0 | n/a |
| Soup, Tortilla, w/chicken | 1 serv. | 320 | 14.0 | 4.0 | 0.0 | 28.0 | n/a |
| No Chicken | 1 serv. | 346 | 14.0 | 4.0 | 0.0 | 28.0 | n/a |
| Tacos | | | | | | | |
| ■ Baja Style Soft Charbroiled Chicken | 1 | 250 | 8.0 | 1.0 | 0.0 | 30.0 | n/a |
| Baja Fish Taco, Breaded Fish | 1 | 320 | 16.0 | 2.5 | 0.5 | 35.0 | n/a |
| Charbroiled Fish | 1 | 300 | 12.0 | 2.0 | 0.0 | 34.0 | n/a |
| Veggie Mix, grilled | 1 serv. | 110 | 0.0 | 0.0 | 0.0 | 12.0 | n/a |
| **Boston Market** | | | | | | | |
| Caesar Salad Entree | 1 | 470 | 40.0 | 9.0 | n/a | 17.0 | 3.0 |
| Chicken | | | | | | | |
| Dark meat, w/skin | 1/4 | 320 | 21.0 | 6.0 | n/a | 2.0 | 2.0 |
| Dark meat, w/o skin | 1/4 | 190 | 10.0 | 3.0 | n/a | 1.0 | 1.0 |
| White meat, w/skin & wing | 1/4 | 280 | 12.0 | 3.5 | n/a | 2.0 | 2.0 |
| Chicken, 1/4, white meat, w/o skin & wing | 1/4 | 170 | 4.0 | 1.0 | 0.0 | 2.0 | 1.0 |
| Chicken Gravy | 1 oz. | 15 | 0.5 | 0.0 | n/a | 2.0 | 0.0 |
| Chicken Noodle Soup | 1 cup | 100 | 4.5 | 1.5 | n/a | 8.0 | 1.0 |
| Chicken Pot Pie | 1 | 750 | 46.0 | 14.0 | n/a | 57.0 | 4.0 |

■ Contains less than 20% fat
n/a Not available

34

| Item | SERVING | CAL-ORIES | FAT GRAMS | SAT. FAT GRAMS | TRANS FAT GRAMS | CARB. GRAMS | SUGAR GRAMS |
|---|---|---|---|---|---|---|---|
| Chicken Salad, Asian grilled, w/dressing & noodles | 1 | 540 | 15.0 | 3.0 | n/a | 57.0 | 45.0 |
| Corn, sweet | 1 serv. | 180 | 4.0 | 0.5 | 0.0 | 30.0 | 13.0 |
| Cornbread | 1 serv. | 120 | 3.5 | 1.0 | n/a | 21.0 | 8.0 |
| ■ Fruit Salad | 1 serv. | 70 | 0.0 | 0.0 | 0.0 | 16.0 | 15.0 |
| Ham, honey glazed | 1 serv. | 210 | 8.0 | 3.0 | n/a | 10.0 | 10.0 |
| Meatloaf & Beef Gravy, Double Sauce, Angus | 2 slices | 580 | 39.0 | 16.0 | n/a | 27.0 | 4.0 |
| ■ Potatoes, garlic dill, low fat | 1 serv. | 130 | 2.5 | 0.0 | 0.0 | 25.0 | 2.0 |
| Potatoes, mashed w/gravy | 1 serv. | 230 | 9.0 | 5.0 | n/a | 32.0 | 4.0 |
| Squash, butternut | 1 serv. | 150 | 6.0 | 4.0 | n/a | 25.0 | 12.0 |
| Stuffing | 1 serv. | 190 | 8.0 | 1.5 | n/a | 27.0 | 5.0 |
| ■ Turkey, breast, w/o skin, low fat, rotisserie | 1 serv. | 170 | 1.0 | 0.0 | 0.0 | 3.0 | 3.0 |
| Turkey Carver Sandwich, w/cheese & sauce | 1 | 690 | 29.0 | 7.0 | n/a | 68.0 | 13.0 |
| ■ Vegetables, steamed | 1 serv. | 30 | 0.0 | 0.0 | 0.0 | 6.0 | 2.0 |
| **Burger King** | | | | | | | |
| Apple Pie | 1 | 300 | 13.0 | 3.0 | 3.0 | 45.0 | 23.0 |
| Cheeseburger | 1 | 350 | 17.0 | 8.0 | 0.5 | 31.0 | 5.0 |
| Chicken Salad, Fire Grilled | 1 | 210 | 7.0 | 3.0 | 0.0 | 12.0 | 3.0 |
| Chicken Sandwich, original | 1 | 560 | 28.0 | 6.0 | 2.0 | 52.0 | 5.0 |
| Chicken Tenders | 8 pieces | 340 | 19.0 | 5.0 | 3.5 | 20.0 | 0.0 |
| Croissan'wich, bacon, egg, & cheese | 1 | 340 | 20.0 | 7.0 | 1.5 | 26.0 | 7.0 |
| w/egg, cheese, & sausage | 1 | 500 | 36.0 | 12.0 | 2.0 | 26.0 | 7.0 |
| Fish Sandwich | 1 | 630 | 30.0 | 5.0 | 1.5 | 69.0 | 9.0 |
| French fries, large | 1 serv. | 500 | 25.0 | 7.0 | 6.0 | 63.0 | 1.0 |
| French fries, small | 1 serv. | 230 | 11.0 | 3.0 | 3.0 | 29.0 | 0.0 |
| French Toast, sticks | 5 pieces | 390 | 20.0 | 4.5 | 4.5 | 46.0 | 11.0 |
| Hamburger | 1 | 310 | 13.0 | 5.0 | 0.5 | 30.0 | 5.0 |
| Hash Browns, medium | 1 serv. | 390 | 25.0 | 7.0 | 8.0 | 38.0 | 0.0 |
| Hash Browns, small | 1 serv. | 230 | 15.0 | 4.0 | 5.0 | 23.0 | 0.0 |
| Milk shake, chocolate, medium | 1 | 600 | 18.0 | 11.0 | 0.0 | 97.0 | 94.0 |
| Vanilla, medium | 1 | 540 | 20.0 | 13.0 | 0.5 | 76.0 | 74.0 |
| Onion Rings, large | 1 serv. | 480 | 23.0 | 6.0 | 5.0 | 60.0 | 7.0 |
| Onion Rings, small | 1 serv. | 180 | 9.0 | 2.0 | 2.0 | 22.0 | 3.0 |
| Whopper | 1 | 700 | 42.0 | 13.0 | 1.0 | 52.0 | 8.0 |
| Whopper w/cheese | 1 | 800 | 49.0 | 18.0 | 2.0 | 53.0 | 9.0 |
| Whopper, double w/cheese | 1 | 1080 | 69.0 | 27.0 | 2.5 | 53.0 | 9.0 |
| Whopper Jr. | 1 | 390 | 22.0 | 7.0 | 0.5 | 31.0 | 5.0 |
| Veggie Burger | 1 | 420 | 16.0 | 3.0 | 3.0 | 46.0 | 7.0 |
| **Carl's Jr.** | | | | | | | |
| Bacon | 2 slices | 45 | 3.5 | 1.5 | n/a | 0.0 | 0.0 |
| Bacon Crispy Chicken Sandwich | 1 | 760 | 38.0 | 11.0 | n/a | 72.0 | 8.0 |

■ Contains less than 20% fat
n/a Not available

| Item | SERVING | CAL-ORIES | FAT GRAMS | SAT. FAT GRAMS | TRANS FAT GRAMS | CARB. GRAMS | SUGAR GRAMS |
|---|---|---|---|---|---|---|---|
| Breakfast Burrito | 1 | 560 | 32.0 | 11.0 | n/a | 37.0 | 1.0 |
| Breakfast Quesadilla | 1 | 390 | 18.0 | 5.0 | n/a | 38.0 | 2.0 |
| Carl's Famous Star Hamburger | 1 | 590 | 32.0 | 9.0 | n/a | 50.0 | 8.0 |
| ■ Charbroiled Chicken Salad | 1 | 330 | 7.0 | 4.0 | n/a | 17.0 | 8.0 |
| Cheeseburger, double, Western Bacon | 1 | 920 | 50.0 | 21.0 | n/a | 65.0 | 14.0 |
| ■ Chicken Sandwich, BBQ, charbroiled | 1 | 370 | 4.0 | 1.0 | n/a | 47.0 | 12.0 |
| Croissant Sunrise Sandwich w/sausage | 1 | 360 | 21.0 | 8.0 | n/a | 28.0 | 5.0 |
| Dressings | | | | | | | |
|   Blue Cheese | 1 serv. | 320 | 35.0 | 6.0 | n/a | 1.0 | 1.0 |
| ■   French, fat free | 1 serv. | 60 | 0.0 | 0.0 | 0.0 | 16.0 | 12.0 |
|   House | 1 serv. | 220 | 22.0 | 4.0 | n/a | 3.0 | 2.0 |
| Fish Sandwich, Carl's Catch | 1 | 560 | 27.0 | 7.0 | n/a | 58.0 | 8.0 |
| French Toast, Dips, w/o syrup | 6 pieces | 450 | 20.0 | 6.0 | n/a | 59.0 | 10.0 |
| ■   Syrup | 1 serv. | 90 | 0.0 | 0.0 | 0.0 | 21.0 | 16.0 |
| Garden Salad | 1 | 120 | 3.0 | 1.5 | n/a | 5.0 | 3.0 |
| ■ Milk | 10 oz. | 150 | 3.0 | 2.0 | 0.0 | 18.0 | 18.0 |
| ■ Potato, baked, w/o margarine | 1 | 280 | 0.0 | 0.0 | 0.0 | 63.0 | 3.0 |
|   w/broccoli & cheese | 1 | 510 | 21.0 | 5.0 | n/a | 71.0 | 4.0 |
|   w/sour cream & chives | 1 | 410 | 14.0 | 4.0 | n/a | 65.0 | 4.0 |
| Scrambled egg breakfast w/bacon | 1 | 760 | 42.0 | 11.0 | n/a | 69.0 | 11.0 |
|   w/sausage | 1 | 900 | 56.0 | 15.0 | n/a | 72.0 | 11.0 |

## Church's Chicken

| Item | SERVING | CAL-ORIES | FAT GRAMS | SAT. FAT GRAMS | TRANS FAT GRAMS | CARB. GRAMS | SUGAR GRAMS |
|---|---|---|---|---|---|---|---|
| Chicken | | | | | | | |
|   Breast w/batter & skin | 1 | 200 | 12.0 | n/a | n/a | 4.0 | 0.0 |
|     No batter & skin | 1 | 145 | 5.5 | n/a | n/a | 1.0 | 0.0 |
|   Crunchy Tenders | 1 piece | 137 | 5.0 | n/a | n/a | 11.0 | 0.0 |
|   Leg w/batter & skin | 1 | 140 | 9.0 | n/a | n/a | 2.0 | 0.0 |
|     No batter & skin | 1 | 118 | 6.2 | n/a | n/a | 1.3 | 0.0 |
|   Thigh w/batter & skin | 1 | 230 | 16.0 | n/a | n/a | 5.0 | 0.0 |
|     No batter & skin | 1 | 180 | 11.0 | n/a | n/a | 3.0 | 0.0 |
|   Wing w/batter & skin | 1 | 250 | 16.0 | n/a | n/a | 8.0 | 0.0 |
|     No batter & skin | 1 | 160 | 7.5 | n/a | n/a | 2.0 | 0.0 |
| Okra | 1 serv. | 210 | 16.0 | 0.0 | 0.0 | 19.0 | <1 |

## Dairy Queen

| Item | SERVING | CAL-ORIES | FAT GRAMS | SAT. FAT GRAMS | TRANS FAT GRAMS | CARB. GRAMS | SUGAR GRAMS |
|---|---|---|---|---|---|---|---|
| Banana Split | 1 | 510 | 12.0 | 8.0 | 0.0 | 96.0 | 82.0 |
| Blizzard, small, Oreo | 1 | 570 | 21.0 | 10.0 | 2.5 | 83.0 | 64.0 |
| Chicken Strip Basket | 6 pieces | 1120 | 60.0 | 11.0 | 15.0 | 102.0 | 9.0 |
| Chocolate Dilly Bar | 1 | 220 | 13.0 | 10.0 | 1.0 | 25.0 | 20.0 |
| French fries, medium | 1 serv. | 380 | 15.0 | 3.0 | 4.5 | 56.0 | <1 |
| Hamburger, homestyle | 1 each | 290 | 12.0 | 5.0 | 0.0 | 29.0 | 5.0 |
| Hot dog | 1 each | 240 | 14.0 | 5.0 | 0.0 | 19.0 | 4.0 |
| Ice cream cone, chocolate, small | 1 | 240 | 8.0 | 5.0 | 0.0 | 37.0 | 25.0 |

■ Contains less than 20% fat
n/a Not available

| Item | SERVING | CAL-ORIES | FAT GRAMS | SAT. FAT GRAMS | TRANS FAT GRAMS | CARB. GRAMS | SUGAR GRAMS |
|---|---|---|---|---|---|---|---|
| Vanilla, small | 1 | 230 | 7.0 | 4.5 | 0.0 | 38.0 | 27.0 |
| ■ Misty Slush, medium | 1 | 290 | 0.0 | 0.0 | 0.0 | 74.0 | 74.0 |
| Peanut Buster Parfait | 1 | 730 | 31.0 | 17.0 | 0.0 | 99.0 | 85.0 |
| Shake, chocolate, medium | 1 each | 760 | 20.0 | 13.0 | 1.0 | 129.0 | 115.0 |
| Soft serve, vanilla | 0.5 cup | 140 | 4.5 | 3.0 | 0.0 | 22.0 | 19.0 |
| Sundae, chocolate, medium | 1 each | 400 | 10.0 | 6.0 | 0.0 | 71.0 | 61.0 |
| **Domino's Pizza** | | | | | | | |
| Classic Hand Tossed Pizza (14" pie) | | | | | | | |
| Cheese | 1 slice | 256 | 8.0 | 3.0 | n/a | 38.0 | 3.0 |
| Green Pepper, Onion, & Mushroom | 1 slice | 263 | 8.0 | 3.0 | n/a | 39.0 | 3.0 |
| Pepperoni | 1 slice | 305 | 12.0 | 5.0 | n/a | 38.0 | 3.0 |
| Crunchy Thin Crust Pizza (14" pie) | | | | | | | |
| Cheese | 1 slice | 188 | 10.0 | 3.5 | n/a | 19.0 | 2.0 |
| Green Pepper, Onion, & Mushroom | 1 slice | 201 | 10.0 | 3.5 | n/a | 21.0 | 3.0 |
| Pepperoni | 1 slice | 237 | 14.5 | 5.5 | n/a | 19.0 | 2.0 |
| Ultimate Deep Dish Pizza (14" pie) | | | | | | | |
| Cheese | 1 slice | 336 | 15.0 | 5.0 | n/a | 41.0 | 4.0 |
| Green Pepper, Onion, & Mushroom | 1 slice | 343 | 15.0 | 5.0 | n/a | 42.0 | 4.0 |
| Pepperoni | 1 slice | 385 | 19.5 | 7.0 | n/a | 41.0 | 4.0 |
| **El Pollo Loco** | | | | | | | |
| Burritos | | | | | | | |
| Bean, Rice, & Cheese | 1 | 528 | 15.0 | 5.0 | n/a | 79.0 | 3.0 |
| Chicken, classic | 1 | 636 | 19.0 | 6.0 | n/a | 81.0 | 3.0 |
| Twice grilled | 1 | 853 | 41.0 | 17.0 | n/a | 62.0 | 3.0 |
| Flame Grilled Chicken | | | | | | | |
| Breast, w/skin | 3.5 oz. | 187 | 7.0 | 2.0 | n/a | 0.0 | 0.0 |
| Breast, no skin | 3.5 oz. | 153 | 4.0 | 1.0 | n/a | 0.0 | 0.0 |
| Leg | 1.8 oz. | 86 | 3.0 | 0.0 | n/a | 0.0 | 0.0 |
| Thigh | 2 oz. | 120 | 7.0 | 2.0 | n/a | 0.0 | 0.0 |
| Wing | 1.5 oz. | 83 | 3.0 | 1.0 | n/a | 0.0 | 0.0 |
| Garden Salad | 1 serv. | 111 | 7.0 | 3.0 | n/a | 8.0 | 3.0 |
| Monterey Pollo Salad | 1 serv. | 258 | 13.0 | 3.0 | n/a | 17.0 | 8.0 |
| ■ Pollo Bowl | 1 | 543 | 10.0 | 1.0 | n/a | 84.0 | 4.0 |
| Taco, chicken, soft | 1 | 237 | 11.0 | 5.0 | n/a | 18.0 | 1.0 |
| Taco, al carbon (chicken) | 1 | 134 | 3.0 | 1.0 | n/a | 18.0 | 0.0 |
| Taquito, chicken | 2 | 370 | 17.0 | 4.0 | n/a | 43.0 | 2.0 |
| ■ Tortilla, corn, 6" | 1 | 210 | 3.0 | 0.0 | n/a | 42.0 | 0.0 |
| Flour, 6.5" | 1 | 330 | 12.0 | 3.0 | n/a | 48.0 | 0.0 |
| Tostada Salad | 1 serv. | 740 | 33.0 | 9.0 | n/a | 83.0 | 9.0 |

■ Contains less than 20% fat
n/a Not available

| Item | SERVING | CAL-ORIES | FAT GRAMS | SAT. FAT GRAMS | TRANS FAT GRAMS | CARB. GRAMS | SUGAR GRAMS |
|---|---|---|---|---|---|---|---|
| **Hardee's** | | | | | | | |
| Apple Turnover | 1 | 290 | 15.0 | 5.0 | n/a | 36.0 | 11.0 |
| Bacon, Egg, & Cheese Biscuit | 1 | 560 | 38.0 | 11.0 | n/a | 37.0 | 4.0 |
| Big Country Breakfast w/Sausage | 1 | 1060 | 64.0 | 15.0 | n/a | 91.0 | 13.0 |
| Biscuit, Cinnamon 'n raisin | 1 | 280 | 12.0 | 3.0 | n/a | 40.0 | 17.0 |
| Biscuit, made from scratch | 1 | 370 | 23.0 | 5.0 | n/a | 35.0 | 3.0 |
| Butter blend | 1 packet | 25 | 3.0 | 1.0 | n/a | 0.0 | 0.0 |
| ■ Strawberry Jam | 1 serv. | 35 | 0.0 | 0.0 | 0.0 | 9.0 | 9.0 |
| Biscuit, w/gravy | 1 serv. | 530 | 34.0 | 8.0 | n/a | 47.0 | 6.0 |
| Chicken Sandwich, charbroiled | 1 | 590 | 26.0 | 7.0 | n/a | 53.0 | 11.0 |
| Cookie, chocolate chip | 1 | 290 | 11.0 | 5.0 | n/a | 44.0 | 26.0 |
| Hamburger | | | | | | | |
| Cheeseburger, 1/3 lb. Hardee's | 1 | 680 | 39.0 | 19.0 | n/a | 52.0 | 11.0 |
| Double Bacon Cheese Thickburger | 1 | 1300 | 96.0 | 40.0 | n/a | 51.0 | 11.0 |
| Monster Thickburger, Hardee | 1 | 1410 | 107.0 | 45.0 | n/a | 47.0 | n/a |
| Thickburger, 1/3 lb. Hardee's | 1 | 850 | 57.0 | 22.0 | n/a | 54.0 | 12.0 |
| Pancake Platter, Hardee | 1 | 300 | 5.0 | 1.0 | n/a | 55.0 | 12.0 |
| Sunrise Croissant w/Bacon | 1 | 450 | 29.0 | 12.0 | n/a | 28.0 | 5.0 |
| **In-N-Out Burger** | | | | | | | |
| Cheeseburger w/mustard & ketchup | 1 | 400 | 18.0 | 9.0 | n/a | 41.0 | 10.0 |
| Double Double w/spread | 1 | 670 | 41.0 | 18.0 | n/a | 39.0 | 10.0 |
| Hamburger w/spread | 1 | 390 | 19.0 | 5.0 | n/a | 39.0 | 10.0 |
| Hamburger, protein style, no bun | 1 | 240 | 17.0 | 4.0 | n/a | 11.0 | 7.0 |
| **Jack-in-the-Box** | | | | | | | |
| Bacon & Cheese Ciabatta Burger | 1 | 920 | 59.0 | 19.0 | 2.0 | 69.0 | 3.0 |
| Double Patty | 1 | 1140 | 79.0 | 28.0 | 3.0 | 69.0 | 7.0 |
| Breakfast Jack | 1 | 290 | 12.1 | 4.6 | 0.4 | 28.6 | 3.9 |
| Breakfast Sandwich, Ultimate | 1 | 574 | 26.9 | 10.1 | 0.8 | 49.0 | 7.6 |
| Cheeseburger, Ultimate | 1 | 1011 | 71.4 | 28.4 | 2.9 | 52.7 | 11.7 |
| Chicken, Jack's Spicy w/cheese | 1 | 697 | 37.1 | 9.6 | 3.0 | 62.4 | 8.5 |
| Chicken Breast Strips | 1 serv. | 630 | 37.3 | 7.7 | 6.0 | 38.2 | 1.8 |
| Chicken Ciabatta | 1 | 510 | 13.0 | 2.5 | 0.0 | 69.0 | 6.0 |
| Chicken Fajita Pita | 1 | 307 | 10.1 | 4.3 | 0.3 | 31.8 | 4.6 |
| Chicken Sandwich | 1 | 402 | 20.8 | 4.5 | 2.3 | 38.5 | 3.6 |
| Chocolate Ice Cream Shake, large | 1 | 1310 | 57.0 | 36.0 | 2.0 | 178.0 | 158.0 |
| Vanilla | 1 | 1140 | 58.0 | 36.0 | 2.0 | 129.0 | 108.0 |
| Fish and Chips | 1 serv. | 887 | 62.8 | 13.0 | 14.3 | 62.3 | 1.7 |
| Fries, Natural Cut, large | 1 serv. | 530 | 25.0 | 6.0 | 7.0 | 69.0 | 1.0 |
| Fries, Seasoned, curly, large | 1 serv. | 550 | 31.0 | 6.0 | 10 | 60.0 | 1.0 |
| Ham & Turkey Pannido Sandwich | 1 | 689 | 33.6 | 10.2 | 0.0 | 57.1 | 4.6 |
| Hamburger | 1 | 310 | 14.0 | 5.5 | 0.9 | 30.3 | 6.1 |
| Jumbo Jack | 1 | 597 | 34.6 | 11.8 | 1.3 | 51.3 | 10.9 |
| Salad, side | 1 | 157 | 8.1 | 2.1 | 0.7 | 15.8 | 3.2 |

■ Contains less than 20% fat
38
n/a Not available

| Item | SERVING | CAL-ORIES | FAT GRAMS | SAT. FAT GRAMS | TRANS FAT GRAMS | CARB. GRAMS | SUGAR GRAMS |
|---|---|---|---|---|---|---|---|
| Sausage w/Croissant Sandwich | 1 | 582 | 39.0 | 13.3 | 3.8 | 36.6 | 4.7 |
| Sourdough Breakfast Sandwich | 1 | 425 | 24.3 | 8.1 | 1.8 | 31.1 | 2.7 |
| Taco | 1 | 160 | 8.0 | 3.0 | 1.0 | 15.0 | 4.0 |
| **KFC** | | | | | | | |
| ■ Baked Beans | 1 serv. | 230 | 1.0 | 1.0 | 0.3 | 46.0 | 22.0 |
| Biscuit | 1 | 190 | 10.0 | 2.0 | 3.5 | 23.0 | 1.0 |
| Chicken | | | | | | | |
| Extra Crispy, w/skin | | | | | | | |
| Breast | 1 piece | 460 | 28.0 | 8.0 | 4.5 | 19.0 | 0.0 |
| ■ no skin or breading | 1 piece | 140 | 3.0 | 1.0 | 0.3 | 0.0 | 0.0 |
| Drumstick | 1 piece | 160 | 10.0 | 2.5 | 1.5 | 5.0 | 0.0 |
| Thigh | 1 piece | 370 | 26.0 | 7.0 | 3.0 | 12.0 | 0.0 |
| Wing | 1 piece | 190 | 12.0 | 4.0 | 2.0 | 10.0 | 0.0 |
| Original Recipe w/skin | | | | | | | |
| Breast | 1 Each | 380 | 19.0 | 6.0 | 2.5 | 11.0 | 0.0 |
| Drumstick | 1 Each | 140 | 8.0 | 2.0 | 1.0 | 4.0 | 0.0 |
| Thigh | 1 Each | 360 | 25.0 | 7.0 | 1.5 | 12.0 | 0.0 |
| Wing | 1 Each | 150 | 9.0 | 2.5 | 1.0 | 5.0 | 0.0 |
| ■ Chicken Sandwich, BBQ | 1 | 300 | 6.0 | 1.5 | 0.5 | 41.0 | 19.0 |
| Chicken Twister | 1 | 670 | 38.0 | 7.0 | 4.0 | 55.0 | 7.0 |
| Cole Slaw | 1 serv. | 190 | 11.0 | 2.0 | 0.3 | 22.0 | 13.0 |
| ■ Corn on the Cob, large | 1 piece | 150 | 3.0 | 1.0 | 0.0 | 26.0 | 10.0 |
| Green Beans | 1 serv. | 50 | 1.5 | 0.0 | 0.0 | 7.0 | 2.0 |
| Macaroni & Cheese | 1 serv. | 400 | 18.0 | 5.0 | 2.5 | 45.0 | 3.0 |
| Mashed Potatoes w/gravy | 1 serv. | 120 | 4.5 | 1.0 | 0.5 | 18.0 | <1 |
| Potato Wedges | 1 serv. | 240 | 12.0 | 3.0 | 4.0 | 30.0 | 0.0 |
| Pot Pie, Chunky Chicken | 1 | 770 | 40.0 | 15.0 | 14.0 | 70.0 | 2.0 |
| **McDonald's** | | | | | | | |
| Apple Pie | 1 | 250 | 11.0 | 3.0 | 4.5 | 34.0 | 13.0 |
| Big Mac | 1 | 560 | 30.0 | 10.0 | 1.5 | 47.0 | 8.0 |
| Biscuit w/Bacon, Egg, & Cheese | 1 | 440 | 24.0 | 8.0 | 5.0 | 36.0 | 3.0 |
| Burrito, Sausage, Breakfast | 1 | 300 | 16.0 | 6.0 | 1.0 | 26.0 | 3.0 |
| Cheeseburger | 1 | 310 | 12.0 | 6.0 | 1.0 | 35.0 | 7.0 |
| Chicken McGrill | 1 | 400 | 16.0 | 3.0 | 0.0 | 38.0 | 7.0 |
| Chicken McNuggets | 4 pieces | 170 | 10.0 | 2.0 | 1.5 | 10.0 | 0.0 |
| Cookies, chocolate chip | 1 pkg. | 270 | 11.0 | 6.0 | 0.0 | 39.0 | 19.0 |
| McDonaldland | 1 pkg. | 250 | 8.0 | 2.0 | 2.5 | 42.0 | 14.0 |
| ■ Dippers, apple | 1 pkg. | 35 | 0.0 | 0.0 | 0.0 | 8.0 | 6.0 |
| Dressings, Newman's Own | | | | | | | |
| Low Fat Vinaigrette | 1 pkg. | 40 | 3.0 | 0.0 | 0.0 | 4.0 | 3.0 |
| Ranch | 1 pkg. | 170 | 15.0 | 2.5 | 0.0 | 9.0 | 4.0 |
| ■ English Muffin | 1 | 150 | 2.0 | 1.0 | 0.0 | 27.0 | 2.0 |
| French Fries, large | 16 oz. | 520 | 25.0 | 5.0 | 6.0 | 70.0 | 0.0 |
| Fruit & Walnut Salad, McDonald's | 1 | 310 | 13.0 | 2.0 | 0.0 | 44.0 | 32.0 |
| ■ Garden Salad w/o dressing | 1 | 15 | 0.0 | 0.0 | 0.0 | 3.0 | 2.0 |

■ Contains less than 20% fat

| Item | SERVING | CAL-ORIES | FAT GRAMS | SAT. FAT GRAMS | TRANS FAT GRAMS | CARB. GRAMS | SUGAR GRAMS |
|---|---|---|---|---|---|---|---|
| Hamburger | 1 | 260 | 9.0 | 3.5 | 0.5 | 33.0 | 7.0 |
| Hash Browns | 1 serv. | 140 | 8.0 | 1.5 | 2.0 | 15.0 | 0.0 |
| Hotcakes w/margarine & syrup | 1 serv. | 600 | 17.0 | 4.0 | 4.0 | 102.0 | 45.0 |
| Ice Cream Cone, reduced fat, vanilla | 1 | 150 | 3.5 | 2.0 | 0.0 | 24.0 | 18.0 |
| McGriddle, Sausage & Cheese | 1 | 560 | 32.0 | 11.0 | 1.5 | 48.0 | 16.0 |
| McMuffin, egg | 1 | 290 | 11.0 | 4.5 | 0.0 | 30.0 | 2.0 |
| Sausage, w/egg | 1 | 450 | 26.0 | 10.0 | 0.5 | 31.0 | 2.0 |
| Sausage, no egg | 1 | 370 | 21.0 | 9.0 | 0.5 | 31.0 | 2.0 |
| Milk, 1% | 1 carton | 100 | 2.5 | 1.5 | 0.0 | 12.0 | 12.0 |
| ■ Parfait, fruit 'n yogurt, w/granola | 1 | 160 | 2.0 | 1.0 | 0.0 | 31.0 | 21.0 |
| ■ Parfait, fruit 'n yogurt, w/o granola | 1 | 130 | 2.0 | 1.0 | 0.0 | 25.0 | 19.0 |
| Quarter Pounder w/cheese | 1 | 510 | 25.0 | 12.0 | 1.5 | 43.0 | 9.0 |
| ■ Sauce, BBQ | 1 pkg. | 45 | 0.0 | 0.0 | 0.0 | 11.0 | 10.0 |
| ■ Honey | 1 pkg. | 50 | 0.0 | 0.0 | 0.0 | 12.0 | 11.0 |
| Hot Mustard | 1 pkg. | 50 | 2.0 | 0.0 | 0.0 | 9.0 | 6.0 |
| ■ Sweet & Sour | 1 pkg. | 50 | 0.0 | 0.0 | 0.0 | 11.0 | 10.0 |
| Scrambled Eggs | 2 | 180 | 11.0 | 4.0 | 0.0 | 5.0 | 0.0 |

**Pizza Hut**

| Item | SERVING | CAL-ORIES | FAT GRAMS | SAT. FAT GRAMS | TRANS FAT GRAMS | CARB. GRAMS | SUGAR GRAMS |
|---|---|---|---|---|---|---|---|
| ■ Apple Dessert Pizza | 1 slice | 260 | 3.5 | 0.5 | 0.5 | 53.0 | 14.0 |
| Bread Stick | 1 | 150 | 6.0 | 1.0 | 0.3 | 20.0 | 4.0 |
| ■ Dipping sauce | 1 serv. | 45 | 0.0 | 0.0 | 0.0 | 9.0 | 6.0 |
| Pizza, Cheese | | | | | | | |
| Full House XL | 1 slice | 280 | 12.0 | 6.0 | 0.5 | 30.0 | 3.0 |
| Personal Pan | 1 | 630 | 27.0 | 12.0 | 1.0 | 71.0 | 14.0 |
| Stuffed Crust, Large | 1 slice | 360 | 13.0 | 8.0 | 0.5 | 43.0 | 8.0 |
| Thin 'N Crispy, Large | 1 slice | 190 | 8.0 | 4.5 | 0.5 | 20.0 | 4.0 |
| Pizza, Lower Fat Chicken, Onion, Pepper, 12" | 1 slice | 170 | 4.5 | 2.0 | 0.3 | 23.0 | 6.0 |
| Pizza, Pepperoni | | | | | | | |
| Full House XL | 1 slice | 290 | 13.0 | 5.0 | 0.3 | 30.0 | 3.0 |
| Personal Pan | 1 | 660 | 30.0 | 12.0 | 1.0 | 70.0 | 14.0 |
| Stuffed Crust, Large | 1 slice | 370 | 15.0 | 8.0 | 0.5 | 42.0 | 8.0 |
| Thin 'N Crispy, Large | 1 slice | 200 | 9.0 | 4.5 | 0.3 | 19.0 | 4.0 |
| Pizza, Personal Pan Supreme | 1 | 750 | 36.0 | 15.0 | 1.0 | 73.0 | 15.0 |

**Popeyes**

| Item | SERVING | CAL-ORIES | FAT GRAMS | SAT. FAT GRAMS | TRANS FAT GRAMS | CARB. GRAMS | SUGAR GRAMS |
|---|---|---|---|---|---|---|---|
| Apple Turnover, Cinnamon | 1 | 250 | 10.0 | 3.0 | n/a | 37.0 | 11.0 |
| Cajun Rice | 1 serv. | 180 | 7.0 | 3.0 | n/a | 23.0 | 1.0 |
| Chicken, Mild | | | | | | | |
| Breast | 1 piece | 510 | 30.0 | 11.0 | n/a | 18.0 | 0.0 |
| Leg | 1 piece | 200 | 12.0 | 4.0 | n/a | 7.0 | 0.0 |
| Strips | 2 pieces | 280 | 13.0 | 5.0 | n/a | 21.0 | 0.0 |
| Thigh | 1 piece | 390 | 27.0 | 9.0 | n/a | 12.0 | 0.0 |
| Wing | 1 piece | 220 | 14.0 | 5.0 | n/a | 10.0 | 0.0 |

■ Contains less than 20% fat
n/a Not available

| Item | SERVING | CAL-ORIES | FAT GRAMS | SAT. FAT GRAMS | TRANS FAT GRAMS | CARB. GRAMS | SUGAR GRAMS |
|---|---|---|---|---|---|---|---|
| Chicken Mild, skinless, breading removed | | | | | | | |
| Breast | 1 piece | 280 | 11.0 | 5.0 | n/a | 7.0 | 0.0 |
| Leg | 1 piece | 110 | 5.0 | 2.0 | n/a | 2.0 | 0.0 |
| Strips | 2 pieces | 200 | 8.0 | 4.0 | n/a | 12.0 | 0.0 |
| Thigh | 1 piece | 220 | 14.0 | 5.0 | n/a | 6.0 | 0.0 |
| Wing | 1 piece | 130 | 7.0 | 3.0 | n/a | 4.0 | 0.0 |
| Chicken Sausage, Jambalaya | 1 serv. | 257 | 13.0 | 3.0 | n/a | 26.0 | 3.0 |
| Chicken Strips, Naked | 3 pieces | 170 | 5.0 | 2.0 | n/a | 2.0 | 0.0 |
| Collard Greens | 1 serv. | 50 | 2.0 | 0.5 | n/a | 7.0 | 1.0 |
| French Fries | 1 serv. | 261 | 12.0 | 5.0 | n/a | 34.0 | 1.0 |
| Popcorn Shrimp | 1 serv. | 280 | 17.0 | 7.0 | n/a | 22.0 | 0.0 |
| Red Beans & Rice | 1 serv. | 340 | 19.0 | 6.0 | n/a | 33.0 | 2.0 |

**Subway**

Sandwiches, 6" 6 g. fat or less

| Item | SERVING | CAL-ORIES | FAT GRAMS | SAT. FAT GRAMS | TRANS FAT GRAMS | CARB. GRAMS | SUGAR GRAMS |
|---|---|---|---|---|---|---|---|
| ■ Chicken Breast, oven roasted | 1 | 330 | 5.0 | 1.5 | 0.0 | 47.0 | 9.0 |
| ■ Ham | 1 | 290 | 5.0 | 1.5 | 0.0 | 47.0 | 8.0 |
| ■ Subway Club | 1 | 320 | 6.0 | 2.0 | 0.0 | 47.0 | 8.0 |
| ■ Sweet Onion Chicken Teriyaki | 1 | 370 | 5.0 | 1.5 | 0.0 | 59.0 | 19.0 |
| ■ Turkey Breast | 1 | 280 | 4.5 | 1.5 | 0.0 | 46.0 | 7.0 |
| ■ Veggie Delite | 1 | 230 | 3.0 | 1.0 | 0.0 | 44.0 | 7.0 |
| Sandwiches, 6" | | | | | | | |
| Italian BMT | 1 | 450 | 21.0 | 8.0 | 0.0 | 47.0 | 8.0 |
| Meatball Marinara | 1 | 560 | 24.0 | 11.0 | 1.0 | 63.0 | 13.0 |
| Subway Melt | 1 | 380 | 12.0 | 5.0 | 0.0 | 48.0 | 8.0 |
| Sandwiches, 6" Double Meat | | | | | | | |
| Cheese Steak | 1 | 450 | 14.0 | 6.0 | 0.0 | 50.0 | 11.0 |
| Seafood Sensation | 1 | 640 | 38.0 | 8.0 | 1.0 | 58.0 | 10.0 |
| Sandwiches, Deli Style | | | | | | | |
| ■ Ham | 1 | 210 | 4.0 | 1.5 | 0.0 | 36.0 | 4.0 |
| Tuna, w/cheese | 1 | 350 | 18.0 | 5.0 | 0.5 | 35.0 | 3.0 |
| ■ Turkey Breast | 1 | 210 | 3.5 | 1.5 | 0.0 | 36.0 | 4.0 |
| Salads | | | | | | | |
| ■ Grilled Chicken & Baby Spinach, no croutons/dressing | 1 | 140 | 3.0 | 1.0 | 0.0 | 11.0 | 4.0 |
| Subway Club | 1 | 160 | 4.0 | 1.5 | 0.0 | 15.0 | 7.0 |
| ■ Veggie Delite | 1 | 60 | 1.0 | 0.0 | 0.0 | 12.0 | 5.0 |
| Salad dressings & condiments | | | | | | | |
| ■ Italian, fat free | 1 serv. | 35 | 0.0 | 0.0 | 0.0 | 7.0 | 4.0 |
| Mayonnaise | 1 serv. | 110 | 12.0 | 3.0 | 0.0 | 0.0 | 0.0 |
| Light | 1 serv. | 50 | 5.0 | 1.0 | 1.0 | 1.0 | 0.0 |
| Ranch | 1 serv. | 200 | 22.0 | 3.5 | 0.0 | 1.0 | 0.0 |

**Taco Bell**

| Item | SERVING | CAL-ORIES | FAT GRAMS | SAT. FAT GRAMS | TRANS FAT GRAMS | CARB. GRAMS | SUGAR GRAMS |
|---|---|---|---|---|---|---|---|
| Burrito, Bean | 1 | 370 | 10.0 | 3.5 | 2.0 | 55.0 | 4.0 |
| Burrito, Beef, Supreme | 1 | 440 | 18.0 | 8.0 | 2.0 | 51.0 | 6.0 |

■ Contains less than 20% fat
n/a Not available

41

| Item | SERVING | CAL-ORIES | FAT GRAMS | SAT. FAT GRAMS | TRANS FAT GRAMS | CARB. GRAMS | SUGAR GRAMS |
|---|---|---|---|---|---|---|---|
| Chalupa, Chicken, supreme | 1 | 370 | 20.0 | 8.0 | 3.0 | 30.0 | 4.0 |
| Beef, supreme | 1 | 390 | 24.0 | 10.0 | 3.0 | 31.0 | 5.0 |
| Steak, supreme | 1 | 370 | 22.0 | 8.0 | 3.0 | 29.0 | 4.0 |
| Gordita, Beef, supreme | 1 | 310 | 16.0 | 7.0 | 0.5 | 30.0 | 7.0 |
| Chicken, supreme | 1 | 290 | 12.0 | 5.0 | 0.0 | 28.0 | 7.0 |
| Steak, supreme | 1 | 290 | 13.0 | 6.0 | 0.5 | 28.0 | 7.0 |
| Nachos, BellGrande | 1 serv. | 780 | 43.0 | 13.0 | 10.0 | 80.0 | 6.0 |
| Pintos & Cheese | 1 serv. | 180 | 7.0 | 3.5 | 1.0 | 20.0 | 1.0 |
| Pizza, Mexican | 1 | 550 | 31.0 | 11.0 | 5.0 | 46.0 | 3.0 |
| Rice, Mexican | 1 serv. | 210 | 10.0 | 4.0 | 1.5 | 23.0 | 1.0 |
| Salad, taco, w/o shell | 1 serv. | 500 | 27.0 | 12.0 | 3.0 | 42.0 | 9.0 |
| Taco | 1 | 170 | 10.0 | 4.0 | 0.5 | 13.0 | 1.0 |
| Taco, Grilled Steak, soft | 1 | 280 | 17.0 | 4.5 | 1.0 | 21.0 | 3.0 |
| Taco, soft, beef | 1 | 191 | 9.1 | 4.1 | 1.0 | 19.1 | 1.8 |
| Tostada | 1 | 250 | 10.0 | 4.0 | 1.5 | 29.0 | 2.0 |
| **Wendy's** | | | | | | | |
| Cheeseburger, Kid's Meal | 1 | 320 | 13.0 | 6.0 | 0.5 | 34.0 | 7.0 |
| Cheeseburger w/bacon, Jr. | 1 | 380 | 18.0 | 7.0 | 0.5 | 34.0 | 6.0 |
| Chicken Nuggets, Kid Size | 4 pieces | 180 | 11.0 | 2.5 | 1.5 | 10.0 | 1.0 |
| ■ Chicken Salad, Mandarin, no dressing | 1 serv. | 170 | 2.0 | 0.5 | 0.0 | 17.0 | 11.0 |
| Chicken Salad, Bacon, Lettuce, Tomato, no dressing | 1 serv. | 330 | 18.0 | 9.0 | 0.0 | 10.0 | 4.0 |
| ■ Chicken Sandwich, Grilled Ultimate | 1 | 360 | 7.0 | 1.5 | 0.0 | 44.0 | 10.0 |
| Chicken Sandwich, homestyle, fillet | 1 | 540 | 22.0 | 4.0 | 1.5 | 57.0 | 8.0 |
| Chicken Fillet Sandwich, Spicy | 1 | 510 | 19.0 | 3.5 | 1.5 | 57.0 | 8.0 |
| Chili, small | 1 serv. | 220 | 6.0 | 2.5 | 0.0 | 23.0 | 6.0 |
| Frosty, small | 1 | 330 | 8.0 | 5.0 | 0.0 | 56.0 | 42.0 |
| ■ Garden Salad, no dressing, side | 1 serv. | 35 | 0.0 | 0.0 | 0.0 | 7.0 | 4.0 |
| Hamburger, Jr. | 1 | 280 | 9.0 | 3.5 | 0.5 | 34.0 | 7.0 |
| ■ Potato, baked, plain | 1 | 270 | 0.0 | 0.0 | 0.0 | 61.0 | 3.0 |
| w/broccoli & cheese | 1 | 440 | 15.0 | 3.0 | 0.0 | 69.0 | 6.0 |
| Salad, taco, supremo, w/o chips | 1 serv. | 380 | 17.0 | 9.0 | 0.5 | 31.0 | 9.0 |
| Salad dressings | | | | | | | |
| Creamy Ranch, reduced fat | 1 packet | 100 | 8.0 | 1.5 | 0.0 | 6.0 | 3.0 |
| ■ French, fat free | 1 packet | 80 | 0.0 | 0.0 | 0.0 | 19.0 | 16.0 |
| Honey mustard, low fat | 1 packet | 110 | 3.0 | 0.0 | 0.0 | 21.0 | 16.0 |
| Spread, Country Crock | 1 serv. | 60 | 7.0 | 1.5 | 0.5 | 0.0 | 0.0 |
| Taco Chips | 1 serv. | 210 | 9.0 | 1.5 | 2.5 | 29.0 | 0.0 |

■ Contains less than 20% fat

| Item | SERVING | CAL-ORIES | FAT GRAMS | SAT. FAT GRAMS | TRANS FAT GRAMS | CARB. GRAMS | SUGAR GRAMS |
|---|---|---|---|---|---|---|---|

## FAST CASUAL

**Applebee's**
Appetizers

| Item | SERVING | CAL-ORIES | FAT GRAMS | SAT. FAT GRAMS | TRANS FAT GRAMS | CARB. GRAMS | SUGAR GRAMS |
|---|---|---|---|---|---|---|---|
| Onion Soup au Gratin | 1 serv. | 150 | 8.0 | n/a | n/a | n/a | n/a |
| Tortilla Chicken Melt | 1 | 480 | 13.0 | n/a | n/a | n/a | n/a |

Desserts

| Item | SERVING | CAL-ORIES | FAT GRAMS | SAT. FAT GRAMS | TRANS FAT GRAMS | CARB. GRAMS | SUGAR GRAMS |
|---|---|---|---|---|---|---|---|
| Berry Lemon Cheesecake | 1 slice | 230 | 7.0 | n/a | n/a | n/a | n/a |
| ■ Chocolate Raspberry Layer Cake | 1 slice | 230 | 3.0 | n/a | n/a | n/a | n/a |

Entrees

| Item | SERVING | CAL-ORIES | FAT GRAMS | SAT. FAT GRAMS | TRANS FAT GRAMS | CARB. GRAMS | SUGAR GRAMS |
|---|---|---|---|---|---|---|---|
| ■ Grilled Shrimp Skewer Salad | 1 | 210 | 2.0 | n/a | n/a | n/a | n/a |
| ■ Grilled Tilapia w/Mango Salsa, w/rice pilaf & vegetables | 1 | 320 | 6.0 | n/a | n/a | n/a | n/a |
| ■ Mesquite Chicken Salad | 1 | 250 | 4.0 | n/a | n/a | n/a | n/a |
| ■ Sizzling Chicken Skillet w/vegetables & whole wheat tortillas | 1 | 360 | 4.0 | n/a | n/a | n/a | n/a |
| Tango Chicken Sandwich w/fresh fruit | 1 | 370 | 9.0 | n/a | n/a | n/a | n/a |
| ■ Teriyaki Steak & Shrimp Skewers w/rice pilaf & vegetables | 1 | 370 | 7.0 | n/a | n/a | n/a | n/a |

**Chili's**

| Item | SERVING | CAL-ORIES | FAT GRAMS | SAT. FAT GRAMS | TRANS FAT GRAMS | CARB. GRAMS | SUGAR GRAMS |
|---|---|---|---|---|---|---|---|
| ■ Guiltless Black Bean Burger | 1 | 650 | 12.0 | 2.0 | n/a | 96.0 | n/a |
| ■ Guiltless Chicken Platter | 1 | 580 | 9.0 | 3.0 | n/a | 85.0 | n/a |
| ■ Guiltless Chicken Sandwich | 1 | 490 | 8.0 | 2.0 | n/a | 63.0 | n/a |
| ■ Guiltless Grill Pita | 1 | 550 | 9.0 | 3.0 | n/a | 70.0 | n/a |
| ■ Guiltless Grill Salmon | 1 | 480 | 14.0 | 3.0 | n/a | 31.0 | n/a |
| ■ Guiltless Tomato Basil Pasta | 1 | 650 | 14.0 | 3.0 | n/a | 107.0 | n/a |

**Olive Garden, Garden Fare Menu**
Dinner entrees

| Item | SERVING | CAL-ORIES | FAT GRAMS | SAT. FAT GRAMS | TRANS FAT GRAMS | CARB. GRAMS | SUGAR GRAMS |
|---|---|---|---|---|---|---|---|
| ■ Capellini Pomodoro | 1 | 644 | 14.0 | n/a | 0.0 | n/a | n/a |
| Chicken Giardino | 1 | 560 | 15.0 | n/a | 0.0 | n/a | n/a |

Kids Entrée

| Item | SERVING | CAL-ORIES | FAT GRAMS | SAT. FAT GRAMS | TRANS FAT GRAMS | CARB. GRAMS | SUGAR GRAMS |
|---|---|---|---|---|---|---|---|
| Grilled Chicken | 1 | 348 | 11.0 | n/a | n/a | n/a | n/a |

Lunch entrees & soup

| Item | SERVING | CAL-ORIES | FAT GRAMS | SAT. FAT GRAMS | TRANS FAT GRAMS | CARB. GRAMS | SUGAR GRAMS |
|---|---|---|---|---|---|---|---|
| ■ Capellini Pomodoro | 1 | 409 | 9.0 | n/a | n/a | n/a | n/a |
| Chicken Giardino | 1 | 408 | 12.0 | n/a | 0.0 | n/a | n/a |
| ■ Linguine alla Marinara | 1 | 340 | 6.0 | n/a | 0.0 | n/a | n/a |
| ■ Minestrone Soup | 1 serv. | 164 | 1.0 | n/a | 0.0 | n/a | n/a |
| Shrimp Primavera | 1 | 483 | 11.0 | n/a | 0.0 | n/a | n/a |

■ Contains less than 20% fat
n/a Not available

| Item | SERVING | CAL-ORIES | FAT GRAMS | SAT. FAT GRAMS | TRANS FAT GRAMS | CARB. GRAMS | SUGAR GRAMS |
|---|---|---|---|---|---|---|---|
| **Ruby Tuesday** | | | | | | | |
| Appetizers | | | | | | | |
| Asian Steamed Dumplings | I serv. | 486 | 21.0 | n/a | n/a | 48.0 | n/a |
| Smart Eating Double Cheese Quesadilla w/Chicken | I plate | 1194 | 97.0 | n/a | n/a | 16.0 | n/a |
| | I plate | 1254 | 98.0 | n/a | n/a | 16.0 | n/a |
| Spicy Buffalo Wings | I plate | 912 | 66.0 | n/a | n/a | 4.0 | n/a |
| Burger Wraps | | | | | | | |
| Smart Eating Grilled Chicken Burger Wrap | I | 470 | 24.0 | n/a | n/a | 10.0 | n/a |
| Smart Eating Turkey Burger Wrap | I | 408 | 17.0 | n/a | n/a | 9.0 | n/a |
| Smart Eating Veggie Burger Wrap | I | 449 | 15.0 | n/a | n/a | 21.0 | n/a |
| Dessert | | | | | | | |
| Low-Carb Cheesecake | I piece | 400 | 32.0 | n/a | n/a | 1.0 | n/a |
| House Specialties | | | | | | | |
| Eat Your Vegetables Platter | I | 673 | 21.0 | n/a | n/a | 73.0 | n/a |
| ■ Smart Eating Pasta Marinara | I | 659 | 10.0 | n/a | n/a | 103.0 | n/a |
| Salads & Soups | | | | | | | |
| Broccoli & Cheese Soup | I serv. | 334 | 27.0 | n/a | n/a | 12.0 | n/a |
| Skinny Chicken Salad | I serv. | 283 | 10.0 | n/a | n/a | 10.0 | n/a |
| Smart Eating Onion Soup | I serv. | 198 | 13.0 | n/a | n/a | 20.0 | n/a |
| White Chicken Chili | I serv. | 218 | 8.0 | n/a | n/a | 22.0 | n/a |
| Side Items & Sauces | | | | | | | |
| ■ Baked Potato, Plain | I | 296 | 2.0 | n/a | n/a | 49.0 | n/a |
| Bleu Cheese Dressing | I serv. | 177 | 19.0 | n/a | n/a | 1.0 | n/a |
| Brown Rice Pilaf, w/Cheese & Tomatoes | I serv. | 223 | 7.0 | n/a | n/a | 34.0 | n/a |
| Creamy Mashed Cauliflower | I serv. | 166 | 11.0 | n/a | n/a | 9.0 | n/a |
| Fresh Steamed Broccoli | I serv. | 129 | 8.0 | n/a | n/a | 5.0 | n/a |
| Light Ranch Dressing | I serv. | 55 | 5.0 | n/a | n/a | 1.0 | n/a |
| ■ Salsa | I serv. | 10 | 0.0 | n/a | n/a | 3.0 | n/a |
| Sauteed Mushrooms | I serv. | 276 | 27.0 | n/a | n/a | 0.0 | n/a |
| Side Caesar Salad | I serv. | 120 | 10.0 | n/a | n/a | 4.0 | n/a |
| ■ Sugar Snap Peas | I serv. | 82 | 0.0 | n/a | n/a | 10.0 | n/a |
| Thai Peanut Sauce | I serv. | 66 | 3.0 | n/a | n/a | 8.0 | n/a |
| Steaks, Seafood & Chicken | | | | | | | |
| Smart Eating Church Street Chicken | I | 523 | 32.0 | n/a | n/a | 0.0 | n/a |
| Smart Eating Creole Catch | I | 312 | 16.0 | n/a | n/a | 0.0 | n/a |
| Smart Eating Grilled Chicken | I | 209 | 5.0 | n/a | n/a | 0.0 | n/a |
| Smart Eating New Orleans Seafood | I | 507 | 31.0 | n/a | n/a | 4.0 | n/a |
| Smart Eating Peppercorn Salmon | I | 287 | 15.0 | n/a | n/a | 0.0 | n/a |
| Smart Eating Petite Sirloin | I | 222 | 8.0 | n/a | n/a | 1.0 | n/a |

■ Contains less than 20% fat
n/a Not available

| Item | SERVING | CAL-ORIES | FAT GRAMS | SAT. FAT GRAMS | TRANS FAT GRAMS | CARB. GRAMS | SUGAR GRAMS |
|---|---|---|---|---|---|---|---|
| Smart Eating Ribeye | 1 | 635 | 44.0 | n/a | n/a | 4.0 | n/a |
| Smart Eating Top Sirloin | 1 | 285 | 11.0 | n/a | n/a | 1.0 | n/a |
| **T.G.I. Friday's** | | | | | | | |
| Appetizers | | | | | | | |
| Buffalo Wings w/dressing | 1 plate | 1010 | 80.0 | 22.0 | n/a | n/a | n/a |
| Tuscan Spinach Dip w/vegetables | 1 plate | 590 | 41.0 | 25.0 | n/a | 17.0 | n/a |
| Dessert | | | | | | | |
| New York Cheesecake | 1 slice | 400 | 25.0 | 15.0 | n/a | 8.0 | n/a |
| Entrees | | | | | | | |
| Barbecue Jack Chicken | 1 | 530 | 10.0 | n/a | n/a | n/a | n/a |
| Bruschetta Grouper | 1 | 500 | 10.0 | n/a | n/a | n/a | n/a |
| Bunless Burgers w/salad & dressing | 1 | 860 | 58.0 | 23.0 | n/a | n/a | n/a |
| Chicken La Boca | 1 | 520 | 27.0 | 13.0 | n/a | n/a | n/a |
| Fire Roasted Salmon w/vegetables | 1 | 440 | 23.0 | 6.0 | n/a | n/a | n/a |
| Grilled Buffalo Chicken salad w/dressing | 1 | 600 | 43.0 | 12.0 | n/a | 10.0 | n/a |
| Key West Grouper w/vegetables | 1 | 300 | 15.0 | 4.0 | n/a | 12.0 | n/a |
| Sante Fe Chicken Salad | 1 | 500 | 10.0 | n/a | n/a | n/a | n/a |
| Sizzling Chicken w/Broccoli | 1 | 620 | 32.0 | 17.0 | n/a | 17.0 | n/a |
| Sizzling NY Strip w/bleu cheese, w/broccoli | 1 | 660 | 38.0 | 18.0 | n/a | 6.0 | n/a |

## FATS & OILS

| Item | SERVING | CAL-ORIES | FAT GRAMS | SAT. FAT GRAMS | TRANS FAT GRAMS | CARB. GRAMS | SUGAR GRAMS |
|---|---|---|---|---|---|---|---|
| Bacon fat | 1 tb. | 125 | 13.8 | 6.3 | 0.0 | 0.0 | 0.0 |
| Beef fat or tallow | 1 tb. | 108 | 12.0 | 6.0 | n/a | 0.0 | 0.0 |
| Butter | | | | | | | |
| Light Whipped, Land O'Lakes | 1 tb. | 35 | 3.5 | 2.5 | 0.0 | 0.0 | 0.0 |
| Stick | 1 tb. | 100 | 11.4 | 7.2 | 0.3 | 0.0 | 0.0 |
| Stick, unsalted | 1 tb. | 100 | 11.4 | 7.2 | 0.3 | 0.0 | 0.0 |
| Whipped | 1 tb. | 68 | 7.7 | 4.8 | 0.2 | 0.0 | 0.0 |
| Butter Blend, Country Morning Soft | 1 tb. | 100 | 11.0 | 2.5 | 2.0 | 0.0 | 0.0 |
| Stick | 1 tb. | 100 | 11.0 | 2.5 | 2.5 | 0.0 | 0.0 |
| Butter, imitation | | | | | | | |
| Molly McButter | 1 tsp. | 5 | 0.0 | 0.0 | 0.0 | 1.0 | 0.0 |
| Chicken fat | 1 tb. | 115 | 12.8 | 3.8 | 0.0 | 0.0 | 0.0 |
| Imitation, Nyafat, Rokeach | 1 tb. | 130 | 15.0 | 2.5 | n/a | n/a | n/a |
| Cooking Spray, Spectrum, brief spray | 1 each | 0 | 0.0 | 0.0 | 0.0 | 0.0 | 0.0 |
| Ghee | 1 tb. | 112 | 12.7 | 7.9 | n/a | 0.0 | 0.0 |
| Lard | 1 tb. | 120 | 13.0 | 5.0 | 0.0 | 0.0 | 0.0 |

■ Contains less than 20% fat
n/a Not available

| Item | SERVING | CAL-ORIES | FAT GRAMS | SAT. FAT GRAMS | TRANS FAT GRAMS | CARB. GRAMS | SUGAR GRAMS |
|---|---|---|---|---|---|---|---|
| Margarine | | | | | | | |
| Benecol Spread | 1 tb. | 80 | 9.0 | 1.0 | 0.0 | 0.0 | 0.0 |
| Benecol Spread, Light | 1 tb. | 50 | 5.0 | 0.5 | 0.0 | 0.0 | 0.0 |
| Fleischmann's Stick, original | 1 tb. | 100 | 11.0 | 2.0 | 2.0 | 0.0 | 0.0 |
| Fleischmann's Soft Tub Spread, original | 1 tb. | 70 | 8.0 | 1.5 | 0.0 | 0.0 | 0.0 |
| Light | 1 tb. | 40 | 4.5 | 0.0 | 0.0 | 0.0 | 0.0 |
| I Can't Believe It's Not Butter, stick | 1 tb. | 90 | 10.0 | 2.0 | 2.5 | 0.0 | 0.0 |
| I Can't Believe It's Not Butter, tub, original | 1 tb. | 80 | 8.0 | 2.0 | 0.0 | 0.0 | 0.0 |
| Land O'Lakes Fresh Buttery Taste Spread | 1 tb. | 80 | 8.0 | 1.5 | 1.5 | 0.0 | 0.0 |
| Parkay, soft, tub | 1 tb. | 60 | 7.0 | 1.5 | 0.0 | 0.0 | 0.0 |
| 60% vegetable oil, squeeze | 1 tb. | 70 | 8.0 | 1.5 | 0.0 | 0.0 | 0.0 |
| ■ Promise fat free, tub | 1 tb. | 5 | 0.0 | 0.0 | 0.0 | 0.0 | 0.0 |
| Shredd's Spread, tub (Country Crock) | 1 tb. | 60 | 7.0 | 1.5 | 0.5 | 0.0 | 0.0 |
| Smart Balance Buttery Spread | 1 tb. | 80 | 9.0 | 2.5 | 0.0 | 0.0 | 0.0 |
| Light | 1 tb. | 45 | 5 | 0.5 | 0.0 | 0.0 | 0.0 |
| Smart Beat Spread | 1 tb. | 22 | 2.0 | 0.0 | 0.0 | 0.0 | 0.0 |
| ■ Smart Beat Squeeze | 1 tb. | 7 | 0.0 | 0.0 | 0.0 | 1.0 | 0.0 |
| Take Control, no trans fat | 1 tb. | 80 | 8.0 | 1.0 | 0.0 | 0.0 | 0.0 |
| Take Control Light, no trans fat | 1 tb. | 45 | 5.0 | 0.5 | 0.0 | 0.0 | 0.0 |
| Oils | | | | | | | |
| Avocado | 1 tb. | 124 | 14.0 | 1.6 | 0.0 | 0.0 | 0.0 |
| Canola | 1 tb. | 120 | 14.0 | 1.0 | 0.0 | 0.0 | 0.0 |
| Coconut | 1 tb. | 117 | 13.6 | 11.8 | 0.0 | 0.0 | 0.0 |
| Corn | 1 tb. | 120 | 13.6 | 1.8 | 0.0 | 0.0 | 0.0 |
| Flaxseed | 1 tb. | 120 | 13.5 | 1.3 | 0.0 | 0.0 | 0.0 |
| Grapeseed | 1 tb. | 120 | 13.6 | 1.3 | 0.0 | 0.0 | 0.0 |
| Olive | 1 tb. | 119 | 13.5 | 1.8 | 0.0 | 0.0 | 0.0 |
| Palm | 1 tb. | 120 | 13.6 | 6.7 | 0.0 | 0.0 | 0.0 |
| Palm Kernel | 1 tb. | 117 | 13.6 | 11.1 | 0.0 | 0.0 | 0.0 |
| Peanut | 1 tb. | 119 | 13.5 | 2.3 | 0.0 | 0.0 | 0.0 |
| Soybean | 1 tb. | 120 | 13.6 | 2.0 | 0.0 | 0.0 | 0.0 |
| Walnut | 1 tb. | 120 | 13.6 | 1.2 | 0.0 | 0.0 | 0.0 |
| Salt pork | 1/2 oz. | 102 | 10.8 | 3.8 | 0.0 | 0.0 | 0.0 |
| Shortening, Crisco | 1 tb. | 110 | 12.0 | 3.0 | 1.5 | 0.0 | 0.0 |
| Spectrum, no trans fat | 1 tb. | 110 | 13.0 | 6.0 | 0.0 | 0.0 | 0.0 |

# FISH & SHELLFISH

The amount of trans fat in all *fried* fish and shellfish depends on the *cooking fat* used.

| Item | SERVING | CAL-ORIES | FAT GRAMS | SAT. FAT GRAMS | TRANS FAT GRAMS | CARB. GRAMS | SUGAR GRAMS |
|---|---|---|---|---|---|---|---|
| ■ Abalone, raw | 3 oz. | 89 | 0.7 | 0.1 | 0.0 | 5.1 | 0.0 |
| Anchovies, canned in oil, drained | 1 oz. | 60 | 2.8 | 0.6 | 0.0 | 0.0 | 0.0 |
| Anchovy paste | 0.5 oz. | 28 | 1.6 | n/a | 0.0 | n/a | n/a |

■ Contains less than 20% fat
n/a Not available

| Item | SERVING | CAL-ORIES | FAT GRAMS | SAT. FAT GRAMS | TRANS FAT GRAMS | CARB. GRAMS | SUGAR GRAMS |
|---|---|---|---|---|---|---|---|
| Arctic char, cooked | 3.5 oz. | 106 | 2.7 | n/a | 0.0 | 0.0 | 0.0 |
| Bass, cooked | | | | | | | |
| Sea | 3.5 oz. | 123 | 2.5 | 0.7 | 0.0 | 0.0 | 0.0 |
| Striped | 3.5 oz. | 123 | 3.0 | 0.6 | 0.0 | 0.0 | 0.0 |
| Bluefish, cooked | 3.5 oz. | 158 | 5.4 | 1.2 | 0.0 | 0.0 | 0.0 |
| Butterfish, cooked | 3.5 oz. | 186 | 10.2 | 3.0 | 0.0 | 0.0 | 0.0 |
| Calamari, fried | 3.5 oz. | 174 | 7.4 | 1.9 | 0.0 | 7.7 | n/a |
| Baked | 3.5 oz. | 138 | 4.7 | 1.0 | 0.0 | 3.7 | n/a |
| Carp, fillet, baked/broiled | 3.5 oz. | 161 | 7.1 | 1.4 | 0.0 | 0.0 | 0.0 |
| Catfish, cooked | | | | | | | |
| Farmed | 3.5 oz. | 151 | 8.0 | 1.8 | 0.0 | 0.0 | 0.0 |
| Wild | 3.5 oz. | 104 | 2.8 | 0.7 | 0.0 | 0.0 | 0.0 |
| Caviar, black and red | 1 tb. | 40 | 2.9 | 0.7 | 0.0 | 0.6 | 0.0 |
| Clams | | | | | | | |
| Canned | 3 oz. | 35 | 0.0 | 0.0 | 0.0 | 2.8 | 0.0 |
| Raw | 3 oz. | 63 | 0.8 | 0.1 | 0.0 | 2.2 | 0.0 |
| Cod, Atlantic, cooked | 3.5 oz. | 104 | 0.9 | 0.2 | 0.0 | 0.0 | 0.0 |
| Dried | 3 oz. | 247 | 2.0 | 0.4 | 0.0 | 0.0 | 0.0 |
| Crab | | | | | | | |
| Blue, canned, drained | 3 oz. | 84 | 1.1 | 0.2 | 0.0 | 0.0 | 0.0 |
| Blue, fresh, cooked | 3 oz. | 101 | 1.0 | 0.0 | 0.0 | 0.0 | 0.0 |
| Dungeness, cooked | 3 oz. | 94 | 1.1 | 0.1 | 0.0 | 0.8 | n/a |
| King, cooked | 3 oz. | 83 | 1.3 | 0.1 | 0.0 | 0.0 | 0.0 |
| Imitation, surimi | 3 oz. | 87 | 1.1 | 0.2 | 0.0 | 8.7 | 0.0 |
| Crayfish, cooked | 3.5 oz. | 81 | 1.2 | 0.2 | 0.0 | 0.0 | 0.0 |
| Dolphin, cooked | 3.5 oz. | 108 | 0.9 | 0.2 | 0.0 | 0.0 | 0.0 |
| Eel, cooked | 3.5 oz. | 231 | 14.6 | 3.0 | 0.0 | 0.0 | 0.0 |
| Fish cake, frozen | 1 each | 231 | 15.3 | 6.0 | n/a | 14.7 | n/a |
| Fish stick, frozen | 1 each | 76 | 3.4 | 0.9 | n/a | 6.7 | 0.7 |
| Flounder, cooked | 3.5 oz. | 116 | 1.5 | 0.4 | 0.0 | 0.0 | 0.0 |
| Gefilte fish | 1 piece | 50 | 1.5 | 0.5 | 0.0 | 3.0 | 0.0 |
| Low sodium | 1 piece | 40 | 1.5 | 0.5 | 0.0 | 1.0 | 0.0 |
| Grouper, cooked | 3.5 oz. | 117 | 1.3 | 0.3 | 0.0 | 0.0 | 0.0 |
| Haddock, cooked | 3.5 oz. | 111 | 0.9 | 0.2 | 0.0 | 0.0 | 0.0 |
| Smoked | 3.5 oz. | 115 | 1.0 | 0.2 | 0.0 | 0.0 | 0.0 |
| Halibut, cooked | 3.5 oz. | 139 | 2.9 | 0.4 | 0.0 | 0.0 | 0.0 |
| Herring, kippered | 3.5 oz. | 215 | 12.3 | 2.8 | 0.0 | 0.0 | 0.0 |
| Pickled | 3.5 oz. | 260 | 17.9 | 2.4 | 0.0 | 9.6 | 0.0 |
| Lingcod, cooked | 3.5 oz. | 108 | 1.4 | 0.3 | 0.0 | 0.0 | 0.0 |
| Lobster | | | | | | | |
| Northern, steamed | 3.5 oz. | 97 | 0.6 | 0.1 | 0.0 | 1.3 | 0.0 |
| Spiny, cooked | 3.5 oz. | 142 | 1.9 | 0.3 | 0.0 | 3.1 | n/a |
| Mackerel, cooked | | | | | | | |
| Atlantic | 3.5 oz. | 260 | 17.7 | 4.1 | 0.0 | 0.0 | 0.0 |
| Jack, canned, drained | 3.5 oz. | 155 | 6.3 | 1.8 | 0.0 | 0.0 | 0.0 |
| Pacific | 3.5 oz. | 199 | 10.0 | 2.9 | 0.0 | 0.0 | 0.0 |
| Mahi mahi, cooked | 3.5 oz. | 108 | 0.9 | 0.2 | 0.0 | 0.0 | 0.0 |

■ Contains less than 20% fat

n/a Not available

| Item | SERVING | CALORIES | FAT GRAMS | SAT. FAT GRAMS | TRANS FAT GRAMS | CARB. GRAMS | SUGAR GRAMS |
|---|---|---|---|---|---|---|---|
| ■ Monkfish, cooked | 3.5 oz. | 96 | 1.9 | 0.5 | 0.0 | 0.0 | 0.0 |
| Mullet, cooked | 3.5 oz. | 149 | 4.8 | 1.4 | 0.0 | 0.0 | 0.0 |
| Mussels, cooked | 3 oz. | 146 | 3.8 | 0.7 | 0.0 | 6.3 | 0.0 |
| ■ Orange roughy, cooked | 3.5 oz. | 88 | 0.9 | 0.0 | 0.0 | 0.0 | 0.0 |
| Oysters, eastern | | | | | | | |
|    Canned, drained | 3 oz. | 59 | 2.1 | 0.5 | 0.0 | 3.3 | 0.0 |
|    Raw | 3 oz. | 50 | 1.3 | 0.4 | 0.0 | 4.7 | n/a |
| Oysters, Pacific, cooked | 3 oz. | 69 | 2.0 | 0.4 | 0.0 | 4.2 | n/a |
| ■ Perch, Lake, cooked | 3.5 oz. | 116 | 1.2 | 0.2 | 0.0 | 0.0 | 0.0 |
| ■ Ocean, cooked | 3.5 oz. | 120 | 2.1 | 0.3 | 0.0 | 0.0 | 0.0 |
| ■ Pike, walleye, cooked | 3.5 oz. | 118 | 1.6 | 0.3 | 0.0 | 0.0 | 0.0 |
| ■ Pollack, Atlantic, cooked | 3.5 oz. | 117 | 1.3 | 0.2 | 0.0 | 0.0 | 0.0 |
| Pompano, cooked | 3.5 oz. | 209 | 12.1 | 4.5 | 0.0 | 0.0 | 0.0 |
| ■ Rockfish, cooked | 3.5 oz. | 120 | 2.0 | 0.5 | 0.0 | 0.0 | 0.0 |
| Sable, smoked | 3.5 oz. | 255 | 20.0 | 4.2 | 0.0 | 0.0 | 0.0 |
| Salmon | | | | | | | |
|    Atlantic, raw | 3.5 oz. | 141 | 6.3 | 1.0 | 0.0 | 0.0 | 0.0 |
|    Atlantic, canned, boneless/ skinless, Kirkland | 3.5 oz. | 112 | 4.2 | 2.1 | 0.0 | 0.0 | 0.0 |
|    Coho, cooked | 3.5 oz. | 177 | 8.2 | 1.9 | 0.0 | 0.0 | 0.0 |
|    Pink, canned | 3.5 oz. | 138 | 6.0 | 1.5 | 0.0 | 0.0 | 0.0 |
|      Wild Alaskan, skinless, canned, Trader Joe's | 3.5 oz. | 105 | 0.9 | 0.0 | 0.0 | 0.0 | 0.0 |
|    Smoked (Lox) | 3.5 oz. | 116 | 4.3 | 0.9 | 0.0 | 0.0 | 0.0 |
|    Sockeye, canned | 3.5 oz. | 152 | 7.3 | 1.6 | 0.0 | 0.0 | 0.0 |
| Sardines | | | | | | | |
|    Atlantic, canned in oil, drained | 3.5 oz. | 206 | 11.4 | 1.5 | 0.0 | 0.0 | 0.0 |
|    Pacific, canned in tomato sauce | 3.5 oz. | 185 | 10.4 | 2.7 | 0.0 | 0.7 | 0.4 |
| Scallops | | | | | | | |
| ■  Bay, raw | 3.5 oz. | 87 | 0.8 | 0.1 | 0.0 | 2.3 | n/a |
| ■  Imitation, surimi | 3 oz. | 84 | 0.4 | 0.1 | 0.0 | 9.0 | n/a |
| ■  Sea, raw | 3.5 oz. | 59 | 0.8 | 0.1 | 0.0 | 2.0 | n/a |
|    Fried | 3.5 oz. | 213 | 8.1 | 2.0 | n/a | 22.3 | 4.1 |
| * ■  Scallops ceviche | 6 oz. | 153 | 1.0 | 0.2 | 0.0 | n/a | n/a |
| * ■  Stir fried | 1 serv. | 182 | 3.3 | 0.4 | n/a | n/a | n/a |
| Shark, fried | 3.5 oz. | 226 | 13.7 | 3.2 | n/a | 6.3 | n/a |
| Shrimp | | | | | | | |
|    Fried, breaded | 3 oz. | 206 | 10.4 | 1.8 | n/a | 9.8 | n/a |
|    Steamed | 3 oz. | 84 | 0.9 | 0.3 | 0.0 | 0.0 | 0.0 |
| Smelt, rainbow, cooked | 3.5 oz. | 123 | 3.1 | 0.6 | 0.0 | 0.0 | 0.0 |
| ■ Snapper, cooked | 3.5 oz. | 127 | 1.7 | 0.4 | 0.0 | 0.0 | 0.0 |
| ■ Sole, cooked | 3.5 oz. | 116 | 1.5 | 0.4 | 0.0 | 0.0 | 0.0 |
| ■ Squid, raw | 3 oz. | 78 | 1.2 | 0.3 | 0.0 | 2.6 | 0.0 |
| Sturgeon, cooked | 3.5 oz. | 134 | 5.1 | 1.2 | 0.0 | 0.0 | 0.0 |
| Sucker, carp, cooked | 3.5 oz. | 161 | 7.1 | 1.4 | 0.0 | 0.0 | 0.0 |

---

■ Contains less than 20% fat
n/a Not available

* See note, page xli

| Item | SERVING | CAL-ORIES | FAT GRAMS | SAT. FAT GRAMS | TRANS FAT GRAMS | CARB. GRAMS | SUGAR GRAMS |
|---|---|---|---|---|---|---|---|
| ■ Sushi, w/vegetables | 3 oz. | 119 | 0.4 | 0.1 | 0.0 | 23.9 | n/a |
| Swordfish, cooked | 3.5 oz. | 154 | 5.1 | 1.4 | 0.0 | 0.0 | 0.0 |
| ■ Tilapia, cooked | 3.5 oz. | 109 | 1.2 | 0.6 | 0.0 | 0.0 | 0.0 |
| Trout, cooked | 3.5 oz. | 189 | 8.4 | 1.5 | 0.0 | 0.0 | 0.0 |
| Rainbow | 3.5 oz. | 149 | 5.8 | 1.6 | 0.0 | 0.0 | 0.0 |
| Rainbow, smoked | 3.5 oz. | 184 | 7.2 | 2.1 | 0.0 | 0.0 | 0.0 |
| Tuna | | | | | | | |
| Bluefin, cooked | 3.5 oz. | 183 | 6.2 | 1.6 | 0.0 | 0.0 | 0.0 |
| Raw | 3.5 oz. | 143 | 4.9 | 1.3 | 0.0 | 0.0 | 0.0 |
| ■ Yellowfin, raw | 3.5 oz. | 107 | 0.9 | 0.2 | 0.0 | 0.0 | 0.0 |
| Tuna, canned, drained | | | | | | | |
| Light, in oil | 3 oz. | 168 | 7.0 | 1.3 | 0.0 | 0.0 | 0.0 |
| ■ Light, in water | 3 oz. | 99 | 0.7 | 0.2 | 0.0 | 0.0 | 0.0 |
| White, in oil | 3 oz. | 158 | 6.9 | 1.1 | 0.0 | 0.0 | 0.0 |
| White, in water | 3 oz. | 109 | 2.5 | 0.7 | 0.0 | 0.0 | 0.0 |
| White, in water, low sodium | 3 oz. | 109 | 2.5 | 0.7 | 0.0 | 0.0 | 0.0 |
| Turbot, cooked | 3 oz. | 104 | 3.2 | n/a | 0.0 | 0.0 | 0.0 |
| Whitefish, cooked | 3 oz. | 146 | 6.4 | 1.0 | 0.0 | 0.0 | 0.0 |
| ■ Smoked | 3 oz. | 92 | 0.8 | 0.2 | 0.0 | 0.0 | 0.0 |
| ■ Whiting, cooked | 3 oz. | 99 | 1.4 | 0.3 | 0.0 | 0.0 | 0.0 |
| Yellowtail, cooked | 3 oz. | 159 | 5.7 | n/a | 0.0 | 0.0 | 0.0 |

## FLOUR & BAKING INGREDIENTS

| Item | SERVING | CAL-ORIES | FAT GRAMS | SAT. FAT GRAMS | TRANS FAT GRAMS | CARB. GRAMS | SUGAR GRAMS |
|---|---|---|---|---|---|---|---|
| Almond paste, packed | 1 tb. | 65 | 3.9 | 0.4 | 0.0 | 6.8 | 5.1 |
| Bisquick mix | ⅓ cup | 163 | 6.1 | 1.6 | 1.5 | 24.7 | 0.7 |
| ■ Reduced fat | ⅓ cup | 152 | 2.5 | 0.5 | 0.5 | 28.3 | 2.0 |
| Carob chips | 1 oz. | 132 | 5.7 | 5.7 | 0.0 | 20.8 | 9.5 |
| Chocolate | | | | | | | |
| Bitter or baking, Hershey | 1 oz. | 158 | 9.6 | 5.9 | 0.0 | 16.2 | 12.8 |
| Bittersweet, Scharffen Berger | 1 oz. | 163 | 9.9 | 6.3 | 0.0 | 14.9 | 9.2 |
| Sweet German, Baker's | 1 oz. | 131 | 7.6 | 4.4 | 0.0 | 17.5 | 15.5 |
| Chocolate chips | | | | | | | |
| Baker's semisweet | 1 oz. | 122 | 7.1 | 4.1 | 0.0 | 18.2 | 16.2 |
| Milk chocolate, Hershey | 1 oz. | 151 | 8.5 | 4.7 | n/a | 17.0 | 15.1 |
| Nestlé Toll House Morsels, semisweet | 1 tb. | 70 | 4.0 | 2.5 | 0.0 | 9.0 | 8.0 |
| Premier White, Hershey | 1 oz. | 151 | 8.0 | 4.9 | 0.0 | 17.3 | 17.0 |
| Special Dark, Hershey | 1 oz. | 151 | 8.5 | 4.7 | 0.0 | 17.0 | 15.1 |
| Cocoa Powder, baking | 1 tb. | 15 | 0.5 | 0.0 | 0.0 | 3.0 | 0.0 |
| ■ Cornmeal, degermed | 1 cup | 489 | 2.4 | 0.6 | 0.0 | 113.7 | 1.4 |
| Flour | | | | | | | |
| ■ Bread | 1 cup | 400 | 0.0 | 0.0 | 0.0 | 88.0 | 0.0 |
| ■ Buckwheat | 1 cup | 402 | 3.7 | 0.8 | 0.0 | 84.7 | 3.1 |
| ■ Cake | 1 cup | 496 | 1.2 | 0.2 | 0.0 | 106.9 | 0.4 |
| ■ Carob | 1 cup | 229 | 0.7 | 0.1 | 0.0 | 91.6 | 50.6 |
| ■ Corn, whole grain | 1 cup | 416 | 4.3 | 0.6 | 0.0 | 87.0 | 0.7 |

■ Contains less than 20% fat
n/a Not available

| Item | SERVING | CAL-ORIES | FAT GRAMS | SAT. FAT GRAMS | TRANS FAT GRAMS | CARB. GRAMS | SUGAR GRAMS |
|---|---|---|---|---|---|---|---|
| ■ Potato | 1 cup | 571 | 0.5 | 0.1 | 0.0 | 132.9 | 5.6 |
| ■ Rice, brown | 1 cup | 574 | 4.4 | 0.9 | 0.0 | 120.8 | n/a |
| ■ Rice, white | 1 cup | 578 | 2.2 | 0.6 | 0.0 | 126.6 | 0.2 |
| ■ Rye | 1 cup | 361 | 1.8 | 0.2 | 0.0 | 79.0 | 1.1 |
| ■ Soybean, defatted | 1 cup | 325 | 5.9 | 0.9 | 0.0 | 29.6 | 17.4 |
| Soybean, full fat | 1 cup | 373 | 18.6 | 2.7 | 0.0 | 25.8 | n/a |
| ■ Spelt, whole grain | 1 cup | 394 | 3.0 | 0.0 | 0.0 | 75.8 | 0.0 |
| ■ Wheat, self-rising | 1 cup | 443 | 1.2 | 0.2 | 0.0 | 92.8 | 0.3 |
| ■ White | 1 cup | 400 | 0.0 | 0.0 | 0.0 | 84.0 | 0.0 |
| ■ Whole wheat | 1 cup | 407 | 2.2 | 0.4 | 0.0 | 87.1 | 0.5 |
| Graham cracker crumbs | ½ cup | 178 | 4.2 | 0.6 | n/a | 32.3 | 13.1 |
| ■ Honey | 1 cup | 1021 | 0.0 | 0.0 | 0.0 | 272.2 | 255.4 |
| ■ Molasses | 1 cup | 951 | 0.3 | 0.1 | 0.0 | 245.1 | 182.0 |
| ■ Splenda | 1 cup | 0.0 | 0.0 | 0.0 | 0.0 | 0.0 | 0.0 |
| Sugar | | | | | | | |
| ■ Brown, packed | 1 cup | 829 | 0.0 | 0.0 | 0.0 | 214.1 | 211.7 |
| ■ Confectioner's/powdered | 1 cup | 467 | 0.1 | 0.0 | 0.0 | 119.5 | 117.5 |
| ■ White, granulated | 1 cup | 774 | 0.0 | 0.0 | 0.0 | 200.0 | 199.8 |
| ■ Syrup, cane or corn | 1 cup | 894 | 0.0 | 0.0 | 0.0 | 237.1 | 234.5 |
| ■ Yeast, active dry | 1 packet | 21 | 0.3 | 0.0 | 0.0 | 2.7 | 0.0 |

## FROZEN FOODS

| | | | | | | | |
|---|---|---|---|---|---|---|---|
| **Beef** | | | | | | | |
| Beef & Broccoli, South Beach Diet | 1 each | 320 | 13.0 | 4.0 | 0.0 | 32.0 | 8.0 |
| Beef Stroganoff, Stouffer's | 1 each | 380 | 17.0 | 5.0 | 0.0 | 33.0 | 4.0 |
| ■ Beef Tips Portobello, Healthy Choice | 1 each | 280 | 8.0 | 3.0 | 0.0 | 28.0 | 16.0 |
| Creamed and chipped beef, Stouffer's | 1 each | 175 | 11.9 | 5.0 | 0.0 | 7.1 | n/a |
| Meatloaf w/potatoes, gravy, & vegetables, Stouffer's | 1 each | 590 | 32.0 | 12.0 | 0.0 | 43.0 | 8.0 |
| ■ Meatloaf w/sauce, vegetables, & apple crisp, Healthy Choice | 1 each | 316 | 5.0 | 2.5 | 0.0 | 52.4 | 17.0 |
| Pepper steak w/rice, Budget Gourmet | 1 each | 230 | 6.0 | 1.5 | n/a | 35.0 | 5.0 |
| Pot Pie, Banquet | 1 each | 400 | 23.0 | 11.0 | 0.0 | 38.0 | 8.0 |
| Pot Roast, Banquet | 1 each | 230 | 10.0 | 4.0 | n/a | 20.0 | 8.0 |
| ■ Pot Roast, Healthy Choice | 1 each | 300 | 6.0 | 2.0 | 0.0 | 41.0 | 24.0 |
| ■ Salisbury Steak, Smart Ones | 1 each | 230 | 5.0 | 2.0 | 0.0 | 32.0 | 4.0 |
| ■ Salisbury steak w/potatoes & vegetables, Lean Cuisine | 1 each | 270 | 8.0 | 4.0 | 0.0 | 27.0 | 10.0 |
| ■ Shepherd's Pie, Amy's | 1 cup | 190 | 3.5 | 1.0 | n/a | 23.0 | 3.0 |
| Stuffed Peppers, Stouffer's | 1 each | 180 | 7.0 | 2.5 | 0.0 | 21.0 | 6.0 |
| Swedish meatballs w/pasta, Lean Cuisine | 1 each | 290 | 8.0 | 3.0 | 0.0 | 33.0 | 5.0 |

■ Contains less than 20% fat
n/a Not available

| Item | SERVING | CAL-ORIES | FAT GRAMS | SAT. FAT GRAMS | TRANS FAT GRAMS | CARB. GRAMS | SUGAR GRAMS |
|---|---|---|---|---|---|---|---|
| **Cheese** | | | | | | | |
| ■ Canneloni, Lean Cuisine | 1 each | 260 | 7.0 | 3.5 | 0.0 | 30.0 | 9.0 |
| Macaroni & Cheese, Lean Cuisine | 1 each | 290 | 7.0 | 4.0 | 0.0 | 42.0 | 8.0 |
| ■ Macaroni & Cheese, Smart Ones | 1 each | 300 | 6.0 | 2.5 | 0.0 | 48.0 | 3.0 |
| Manicotti, Healthy Choice | 1 each | 300 | 9.0 | 3.0 | n/a | 40.0 | 14.0 |
| Mozzarella Sticks, TGIF | 1 serv. | 100 | 6.0 | 2.0 | n/a | 9.0 | 1.0 |
| Quesadilla, Whole Foods | 3 each | 590 | 32.0 | 18.0 | 0.0 | 46.0 | 2.0 |
| **Chicken** | | | | | | | |
| ■ Asian Style Pot Sticker, Lean Cuisine | 1 package | 320 | 6.0 | 2.0 | 0.0 | 55.0 | 11.0 |
| Biryani, Ethnic Gourmet | 1 each | 410 | 12.0 | 1.5 | 0.0 | 57.0 | 7.0 |
| ■ Cacciatore, w/pasta & vegetables, Healthy Choice | 1 each | 266 | 4.0 | 1.0 | 0.0 | 35.9 | 9.9 |
| Chow Mein, Lean Cuisine | 1 each | 190 | 2.5 | 0.5 | 0.0 | 29.0 | 4.0 |
| Cordon Bleu, Barber | 1 piece | 370 | 23.0 | 7.0 | 0.0 | 14.0 | 1.0 |
| ■ Enchilada w/beans & rice, El Charrito | 1 each | 400 | 8.0 | 2.5 | n/a | 67.0 | 7.0 |
| w/sauce, rice, corn, & compote, Healthy Choice | 1 each | 298 | 6.7 | 3.1 | 0.0 | 46.0 | 8.0 |
| Fajita kit, Tyson | 1 each | 129 | 3.3 | 0.8 | 0.0 | 17.4 | n/a |
| Fried, Banquet | 1 each | 470 | 27.0 | 9.0 | 1.0 | 35.0 | 4.0 |
| No skin, Banquet | 6 oz. | 440 | 26.0 | 6.0 | 0.0 | 14.0 | 2.0 |
| Glazed, w/rice pilaf & green beans, Lean Cuisine | 1 each | 240 | 6.0 | 1.0 | 0.0 | 25.0 | 7.0 |
| Grilled chicken in wine sauce, Lean Cuisine | 1 each | 160 | 5.0 | 1.0 | 0.0 | 15.0 | 4.0 |
| ■ Honey Dijon, Smart Ones | 1 each | 210 | 3.5 | 1.0 | n/a | 38.0 | 9.0 |
| Korma, Ethnic Gourmet | 1 each | 360 | 10.0 | 2.0 | n/a | 34.0 | 5.0 |
| Lemon, Lean Cuisine | 1 each | 290 | 7.0 | 1.5 | 0.0 | 45.0 | 8.0 |
| Lemongrass, Lean Cuisine | 1 each | 240 | 6.0 | 3.5 | 0.0 | 29.0 | 4.0 |
| ■ Mediterranean, Spa/Lean Cuisine | 1 each | 240 | 3.5 | 0.5 | 0.0 | 35.0 | 7.0 |
| Mesquite BBQ, w/corn & potato, Tyson | 1 each | 321 | 7.8 | 2.6 | n/a | 45.0 | n/a |
| Nuggets, Banquet | 6 pieces | 270 | 19.0 | 4.0 | 0.0 | 12.0 | 2.0 |
| ■ Pad Thai, Ethnic Gourmet | 1 each | 430 | 8.0 | 1.5 | n/a | 71.0 | 20.0 |
| Parmesan, Butterball | 1 piece | 200 | 7.0 | 3.0 | n/a | 16.0 | 5.0 |
| Healthy Choice | 1 each | 330 | 8.0 | 3.0 | n/a | 46.0 | 23.0 |
| Pasta bake, Stouffer's | 1 each | 350 | 13.0 | 4.0 | n/a | 37.0 | 4.0 |
| ■ Patty, fat free, Banquet | 1 each | 100 | 0.0 | 0.0 | 0.0 | 15.0 | 3.0 |
| Peanut Satay, Ethnic Gourmet | 1 each | 410 | 12.0 | 2.0 | n/a | 51.0 | 8.0 |
| Peanut Sauce, Spa/Lean Cuisine | 1 each | 280 | 7.0 | 1.5 | 0.0 | 32.0 | 6.0 |
| Pot Pie, Stouffer's | 1 each | 580 | 35.0 | 15.0 | 0.0 | 50.0 | 9.0 |
| Healthy Choice | 1 each | 310 | 7.0 | 2.5 | 0.0 | 40.0 | 15.0 |

■ Contains less than 20% fat
n/a Not available

51

| Item | SERVING | CAL-ORIES | FAT GRAMS | SAT. FAT GRAMS | TRANS FAT GRAMS | CARB. GRAMS | SUGAR GRAMS |
|---|---|---|---|---|---|---|---|
| ■ Roasted w/mushrooms, rice, & broccoli, Lean Cuisine | 1 each | 330 | 5.0 | 1.0 | n/a | 49.0 | 5.0 |
| Sausage w/fresh spinach & feta, Hans' All Natural, Costco | 1 link | 150 | 8.0 | 2.5 | 0.0 | 1.0 | 0.0 |
| Sesame Chicken, Stouffer's Corner Bistro | 1 each | 510 | 15.0 | 2.5 | 0.0 | 72.0 | 19.0 |
| ■ Sweet & Sour, Lean Cuisine | 1 each | 290 | 2.5 | 0.5 | 0.0 | 53.0 | 20.0 |
| Tandoori w/spinach, Ethnic Gourmet | 1 each | 330 | 10.0 | 2.0 | n/a | 39.0 | 3.0 |
| ■ Thai Style, Lean Cuisine | 1 each | 230 | 4.0 | 2.0 | 0.0 | 30.0 | 8.0 |
| w/broccoli & cheese stuffing, Barber | 1 piece | 360 | 19.0 | 6.0 | 0.0 | 20.0 | 3.0 |

**Kosher Foods**
**Appetizers**

| Item | SERVING | CAL-ORIES | FAT GRAMS | SAT. FAT GRAMS | TRANS FAT GRAMS | CARB. GRAMS | SUGAR GRAMS |
|---|---|---|---|---|---|---|---|
| Challah, ready to bake, Kineret | 1 slice | 150 | 4.0 | 1.0 | 0.0 | 25.0 | 4.0 |
| ■ Chili, vegetarian, Tabatchnick | 1 cup | 180 | 3.5 | 0.0 | 0.0 | 28.0 | 3.0 |
| Egg Rolls, cocktail size, Barney's | 3 each | 160 | 6.0 | 1.0 | n/a | 22.0 | 1.0 |
| ■ Knish, Potato, Cohen's | 1 each | 150 | 3.0 | 0.0 | 0.0 | 29.0 | 4.0 |

**Entrees**

| Item | SERVING | CAL-ORIES | FAT GRAMS | SAT. FAT GRAMS | TRANS FAT GRAMS | CARB. GRAMS | SUGAR GRAMS |
|---|---|---|---|---|---|---|---|
| Bow Ties with Kasha, Cohen's | ¾ cup | 160 | 6.0 | 1.0 | 0.0 | 22.0 | 0.0 |
| Broccoli Soufflé, Melrose Made Gourmet | 1 each | 130 | 7.0 | 1.0 | 0.0 | 12.0 | 2.0 |
| Chicken Nuggets, Empire | 5 each | 230 | 7.0 | 1.5 | 0.0 | 26.0 | 0.0 |
| Cod Sticks, Lightly Breaded, Trader Joe's | 6 each | 170 | 8.0 | 1.0 | n/a | 12.0 | 2.0 |
| Enchilada, Bean & Vegetable, Amy's | 1 each | 180 | 6.0 | 0.5 | 0.0 | 26.0 | 2.0 |
| Potato Kugel Soufflé, Melrose Made Gourmet | 1 each | 230 | 15.0 | 2.5 | 0.0 | 20.0 | 2.0 |
| ■ Potato & Onion Pierogie, Mrs. T's | 3 each | 170 | 2.0 | 0.0 | 0.0 | 33.0 | 1.0 |
| Potato Pancakes, Golden's | 2 each | 140 | 6.0 | 0.0 | 0.0 | 20.0 | 4.0 |
| Spanakopita, Apollo | 2 each | 170 | 10.0 | 3.0 | 1.5 | 17.0 | 1.0 |
| Spinach & Cheese Fillo pie, Fillo Factory | ⅕ pie | 240 | 10.0 | 4.5 | 0.0 | 27.0 | 1.0 |
| Sweet & Sour Chicken Breast w/rice and vegetable, Empire Culinary | 1 each | 290 | 7.0 | 1.5 | n/a | 28.0 | 7.0 |
| Sweet Potato Pancakes, Golden | 2 each | 160 | 8.0 | 1.0 | 0.0 | 20.0 | 8.0 |
| Turkey Meatloaf w/vegetable, Empire Culinary Cuisine | 1 each | 330 | 14.0 | 3.5 | n/a | 31.0 | 5.0 |
| Zucchini Pancakes, Golden's | 2 each | 140 | 6.0 | 1.0 | 0.0 | 16.0 | 2.0 |

**Soups**

| Item | SERVING | CAL-ORIES | FAT GRAMS | SAT. FAT GRAMS | TRANS FAT GRAMS | CARB. GRAMS | SUGAR GRAMS |
|---|---|---|---|---|---|---|---|
| Chicken, Noodles, and Dumplings, Tabatchnick | 1 cup | 150 | 6.0 | 1.0 | 0.0 | 19.0 | 1.0 |

■ Contains less than 20% fat
n/a Not available

| Item | SERVING | CAL-ORIES | FAT GRAMS | SAT. FAT GRAMS | TRANS FAT GRAMS | CARB. GRAMS | SUGAR GRAMS |
|---|---|---|---|---|---|---|---|
| ■ Minestrone, Tabatchnick | 1 cup | 120 | 1.0 | 0.0 | 0.0 | 24.0 | 3.0 |
| ■ Split Pea, Tabatchnick | 1 cup | 140 | 0.0 | 0.0 | 0.0 | 34.0 | 0.0 |
| **Pasta** | | | | | | | |
| Fettucine Alfredo, Stouffer's | 1 each | 540 | 23.0 | 12.0 | 0.0 | 64.0 | 7.0 |
| ■ Healthy Choice | 1 each | 240 | 5.0 | 2.5 | 0.0 | 37.0 | 4.0 |
| Lasagna | | | | | | | |
| w/meat sauce, Stouffer's | 1 each | 370 | 14.0 | 8.0 | 0.0 | 35.0 | 5.0 |
| Budget Gourmet | 1 each | 300 | 9.0 | 3.0 | 0.0 | 40.0 | 5.0 |
| Budget Gourmet, low fat | 1 each | 250 | 7.0 | 3.0 | 0.0 | 34.0 | 6.0 |
| ■ Healthy Choice | 1 each | 420 | 9.0 | 3.0 | 0.0 | 59.0 | 14.0 |
| Florentine, Smart Ones | 1 each | 290 | 8.0 | 4.5 | 0.0 | 36.0 | 3.0 |
| ■ Garden Vegetable, Cedarlane | 1 serv. | 180 | 3.0 | 2.0 | 0.0 | 26.0 | 2.0 |
| w/vegetables, Amy's | 1 each | 290 | 9.0 | 4.0 | 0.0 | 41.0 | 7.0 |
| Lean Cuisine | 1 each | 260 | 7.0 | 3.5 | 0.0 | 33.0 | 9.0 |
| w/tofu & vegetables, Amy's | 1 each | 300 | 10.0 | 1.5 | 0.0 | 41.0 | 6.0 |
| w/mozzarella, Budget Gourmet | 1 each | 300 | 8.0 | 3.0 | 0.0 | 45.0 | 4.0 |
| Penne, w/Italian sausage & sauce, low fat, Budget Gourmet | 1 each | 270 | 6.0 | 1.5 | 0.0 | 46.0 | 4.0 |
| Spaghetti Marinara, low fat, Budget Gourmet | 1 each | 270 | 6.0 | 1.5 | 0.0 | 45.0 | 5.0 |
| **Pizza** | | | | | | | |
| Cheese | | | | | | | |
| Amy's | ⅓ pizza | 290 | 1.0 | 1.0 | 0.0 | 37.0 | 3.0 |
| Extra cheese, for one, Tombstone | 1 each | 400 | 18.0 | 9.0 | 2.0 | 41.0 | 5.0 |
| French Bread, Marie Callender's | 1 each | 360 | 15.0 | 7.0 | 0.0 | 41.0 | 3.0 |
| Soy cheese, Amy's | ⅓ pizza | 310 | 12.0 | 4.0 | 0.0 | 38.0 | 4.0 |
| Pepperoni | | | | | | | |
| French bread, Lean Cuisine | 1 piece | 310 | 9.0 | 3.5 | 0.0 | 43.0 | 6.0 |
| Smart Ones | 1 pizza | 390 | 11.0 | 3.5 | 0.0 | 50.0 | 8.0 |
| Tombstone | ¼ pizza | 380 | 19.0 | 8.0 | 0.0 | 36.0 | 5.0 |
| Vegetable | | | | | | | |
| DiGiorno, w/chicken | ½ piece | 290 | 8.0 | 3.5 | 0.0 | 38.0 | 4.0 |
| French Bread, Stouffer's | 1 each | 350 | 12.0 | 5.0 | 0.0 | 48.0 | 5.0 |
| ■ Healthy Choice | 1 each | 280 | 4.0 | 1.5 | 0.0 | 44.0 | 8.0 |
| Less fat, for one, Tombstone | 1 each | 360 | 9.0 | 4.0 | n/a | 48.0 | 11.0 |
| Roasted veggies, no cheese, Amy's | ⅓ pizza | 276 | 9.0 | 1.5 | 0.0 | 42.0 | 5.0 |
| **Pockets & Sandwiches** | | | | | | | |
| Beef shredded w/cheddar cheese, Ore-Ida | 1 each | 430 | 19.0 | 7.0 | n/a | 45.0 | 2.0 |

■ Contains less than 20% fat
n/a Not available

53

| Item | SERVING | CAL-ORIES | FAT GRAMS | SAT. FAT GRAMS | TRANS FAT GRAMS | CARB. GRAMS | SUGAR GRAMS |
|---|---|---|---|---|---|---|---|
| ■ Breakfast Burrito, Amy's | 1 each | 250 | 7.0 | 0.5 | 0.0 | 38.0 | 4.0 |
| Burrito, bean & rice, Amy's | 1 each | 280 | 6.0 | 0.5 | 0.0 | 48.0 | 2.0 |
| Burrito Grande w/Chili Verde Sauce, Cedarlane | ½ each | 230 | 10.0 | 4.0 | 0.0 | 27.0 | 3.0 |
| Cheeseburger, White Castle | 2 each | 310 | 17.0 | 9.0 | n/a | 23.0 | 0.0 |
| Chicken Pannini, Lean Cuisine | 1 each | 280 | 8.0 | 3.5 | 0.0 | 32.0 | 3.0 |
| Ham & Cheese, Hot Pocket | 1 each | 310 | 13.0 | 5.0 | 0.0 | 38.4 | 7.0 |
| ■ Philly beef steak sandwich, Healthy Choice | 1 each | 310 | 5.0 | 1.5 | n/a | 50.0 | 10.0 |
| Pizza, veggie, w/soy cheese, Amy's | 1 each | 260 | 8.0 | 0.5 | 0.0 | 39.0 | 4.0 |
| Roasted vegetable, Amy's | 1 each | 220 | 8.0 | 1.5 | 0.0 | 35.0 | 5.0 |
| Spinach w/feta, Amy's | ⅓ each | 310 | 12.0 | 4.5 | 0.0 | 47.0 | 6.0 |
| Turkey, broccoli & cheese, Lean Pocket | 1 each | 230 | 7.0 | 3.0 | 0.0 | 30.0 | 12.0 |
| Turkey, Ham, & Cheddar, Lean Pocket | 1 each | 280 | 7.0 | 3.0 | 0.0 | 44.0 | 8.0 |
| Vegetarian Loaf, Amy's | 1 each | 280 | 7.0 | 1.0 | 0.0 | 47.0 | 6.0 |
| ■ Veggie Wrap w/couscous and vegetables, Cedarlane | 1 each | 220 | 3.0 | 0.0 | 0.0 | 36.0 | 2.0 |
| **Seafood** | | | | | | | |
| Alaska Pollack and Macaroni, Stouffer's | 1 each | 430 | 18.0 | 6.0 | 0.0 | 47.0 | 5.0 |
| ■ Baked fish w/pasta shells, vegetables, & cheese sauce, Lean Cuisine | 1 each | 290 | 6.0 | 3.0 | 0.0 | 40.0 | 6.0 |
| Clams, fried, Mrs. Paul's | 3 oz. | 280 | 14.5 | n/a | n/a | 29.0 | 3.0 |
| Egg roll, shrimp, mini, La Choy | 6 each | 190 | 6.0 | 1.5 | n/a | 28.0 | 3.0 |
| Egg roll, vegetable, w/lobster, mini, La Choy | 6 each | 190 | 7.0 | 1.5 | n/a | 27.0 | 3.0 |
| ■ Flounder, fillet, natural, Van de Kamp's | 1 each | 110 | 2.0 | 0.0 | 0.0 | 0.0 | 0.0 |
| Lemon Pepper Fish, Lean Cuisine | 1 each | 220 | 6.0 | 2.0 | 0.0 | 20.0 | 5.0 |
| Salmon w/Basil, Spa/Lean Cuisine | 1 each | 260 | 8.0 | 2.5 | 0.0 | 31.0 | 4.0 |
| Seafood Scampi, Corner Bistro | 1 each | 410 | 12.0 | 5.0 | 0.0 | 56.0 | 5.0 |
| Shrimp w/Lemon & Garlic, Lean Cuisine | 1 each | 280 | 7.0 | 3.5 | 0.0 | 38.0 | 3.0 |
| ■ Tuna Noodle au Gratin, Smart Ones | 1 each | 250 | 4.5 | 1.5 | 0.0 | 37.0 | 5.0 |
| **Turkey** | | | | | | | |
| ■ Breast, traditional, Healthy Choice | 1 each | 290 | 4.5 | 2.0 | 0.0 | 40.0 | 20.0 |
| Breast, w/potatoes & vegetables, Stouffer's | 1 each | 460 | 16.0 | 5.0 | 0.0 | 55.0 | 6.0 |
| Dinner w/gravy, dressing, mashed potatoes, & corn, Banquet | 1 each | 280 | 9.9 | 2.5 | n/a | 34.0 | 6.6 |

■ Contains less than 20% fat

| Item | SERVING | CAL-ORIES | FAT GRAMS | SAT. FAT GRAMS | TRANS FAT GRAMS | CARB. GRAMS | SUGAR GRAMS |
|---|---|---|---|---|---|---|---|
| Dinner, mostly white meat, Hungry Man | 1 each | 510 | 15.0 | 4.0 | n/a | 64.0 | 22.0 |
| Divan, bowl, Healthy Choice | 1 each | 250 | 6.0 | 2.0 | n/a | 31.0 | 7.0 |
| Escalloped noodles w/white turkey & sauce, Budget Gourmet | 1 each | 320 | 15.0 | 5.0 | n/a | 35.0 | 5.0 |
| ■ Glazed, low fat, Budget Gourmet | 1 each | 260 | 5.0 | 2.0 | n/a | 43.0 | 4.0 |
| ■ Glazed tenderloin, w/stuffing & potato, Lean Cuisine | 1 each | 260 | 4.5 | 1.0 | 0.0 | 41.0 | 20.0 |
| Pot Pie, Marie Callendar | ½ pie | 510 | 31.0 | 8.0 | 0.0 | 43.0 | 6.0 |
| Stouffer's | ½ pie | 580 | 35.0 | 15.0 | 0.0 | 50.0 | 9.0 |
| ■ Roast Medallions, Smart Ones | 1 each | 200 | 10.0 | 2.0 | 0.0 | 11.0 | 3.0 |
| Tetrazzini, Stouffer's | 1 each | 380 | 20.0 | 8.0 | 0.0 | 32.0 | 6.0 |
| **Pork &Veal** | | | | | | | |
| Pork | | | | | | | |
| Pork w/pecans & green beans, South Beach Diet | 1 each | 260 | 13.0 | 3.5 | 0.0 | 13.0 | 5.0 |
| ▬ Honey roasted w/potatoes, carrots, & peppers, Lean Cuisine | 1 each | 240 | 5.0 | 2.0 | 0.0 | 31.0 | 10.0 |
| Ribs, no bone, Banquet | 1 each | 400 | 19.0 | 8.0 | n/a | 40.0 | 22.0 |
| ■ w/Cherry Sauce, Spa/Lean Cuisine | 1 each | 260 | 5.0 | 2.0 | 0.0 | 38.0 | 12.0 |
| Veal | | | | | | | |
| Parmigiana, w/tomato sauce, Morton | 1 each | 290 | 15.0 | 4.5 | 0.0 | 30.0 | 8.0 |
| w/spaghetti & vegetables, Stouffer's | 1 each | 530 | 17.0 | 4.5 | 0.0 | 66.0 | 14.0 |
| **Vegetarian** | | | | | | | |
| Brown rice & vegetable bowl, Amy's | 1 each | 240 | 8.0 | 1.0 | 0.0 | 36.0 | 7.0 |
| Chik nuggets, Morningstar Farms | 4 pieces | 190 | 7.0 | 1.0 | 0.0 | 18.0 | 1.0 |
| Corn dogs, veggie, Morningstar Farms | 1 each | 150 | 4.0 | 0.5 | 0.0 | 22.0 | 4.0 |
| Eggplant Parmesan, Cedarlane | 1 serv. | 160 | 8.0 | 3.0 | 0.0 | 16.0 | 3.0 |
| Egg Roll, veggie, w/rice, Lean Cuisine | 1 each | 310 | 5.0 | 1.0 | 0.0 | 60.0 | 17.0 |
| ■ Enchilada, Garden Vegetable, low fat, Cedarlane | 1 piece | 140 | 3.0 | 1.5 | 0.0 | 20.0 | 4.0 |
| Pot pie, vegetable, nondairy, Amy's | 1 each | 360 | 13.0 | 1.5 | n/a | 50.0 | 3.0 |
| Vegetable Burgers: Boca Original Vegan | 1 each | 70 | 0.5 | 0.0 | 0.0 | 6.0 | 0.0 |

■ Contains less than 20% fat
n/a Not available

| Item | SERVING | CAL-ORIES | FAT GRAMS | SAT. FAT GRAMS | TRANS FAT GRAMS | CARB. GRAMS | SUGAR GRAMS |
|---|---|---|---|---|---|---|---|
| ■ Spicy Black Bean, Morningstar Farms | 1 each | 115 | 0.8 | 0.2 | 0.0 | 15.2 | 1.4 |
| ■ Veggie Loaf | 1 each | 280 | 7.0 | 1.0 | 0.0 | 47.0 | 6.0 |

## FRUITS

| Item | SERVING | CAL-ORIES | FAT GRAMS | SAT. FAT GRAMS | TRANS FAT GRAMS | CARB. GRAMS | SUGAR GRAMS |
|---|---|---|---|---|---|---|---|
| ■ Apples, fresh | 1 | 72 | 0.2 | 0.0 | 0.0 | 19.1 | 14.3 |
| Chips, Seneca | 1 oz. | 140 | 7.0 | 0.5 | 0.0 | 20.0 | 11.0 |
| ■ Dried rings | 1 | 16 | 0.0 | 0.0 | 0.0 | 4.2 | 3.7 |
| Applesauce | | | | | | | |
| ■ Sweetened | 1/2 cup | 97 | 0.2 | 0.0 | 0.0 | 25.4 | 21.0 |
| ■ Unsweetened | 1/2 cup | 52 | 0.1 | 0.0 | 0.0 | 13.8 | 12.3 |
| ■ Apricots, fresh | 1 | 17 | 0.1 | 0.0 | 0.0 | 3.9 | 3.2 |
| ■ Canned, packed in juice | 1/2 cup | 59 | 0.1 | 0.0 | 0.0 | 15.1 | 13.1 |
| ■ Canned, in heavy syrup | 1/2 cup | 107 | 0.1 | 0.0 | 0.0 | 27.7 | 25.6 |
| ■ Dried, uncooked | 1 | 8 | 0.0 | 0.0 | 0.0 | 2.2 | 1.9 |
| Avocado | | | | | | | |
| California | 1 | 289 | 26.7 | 3.7 | 0.0 | 15.0 | 0.5 |
| Florida | 1 | 365 | 30.6 | 6.0 | 0.0 | 23.8 | 7.1 |
| ■ Banana, fresh | 1 | 105 | 0.4 | 0.1 | 0.0 | 27.0 | 14.4 |
| ■ Blackberries, fresh | 1/2 cup | 31 | 0.4 | 0.0 | 0.0 | 6.9 | 3.3 |
| ■ Frozen, unsweetened, | 1/2 cup | 48 | 0.3 | 0.0 | 0.0 | 11.8 | 8.1 |
| ■ Blueberries, fresh | 1/2 cup | 41 | 0.2 | 0.0 | 0.0 | 10.5 | 7.2 |
| ■ Frozen, unsweetened | 1/2 cup | 40 | 0.5 | 0.0 | 0.0 | 9.4 | 6.6 |
| ■ Boysenberries, fresh | 1/2 cup | 31 | 0.4 | 0.0 | 0.0 | 6.9 | 3.3 |
| ■ Breadfruit, fresh | 1 | 396 | 0.9 | 0.2 | 0.0 | 104.1 | 42.2 |
| ■ Cantaloupe, fresh | 1/4 | 47 | 0.3 | 0.1 | 0.0 | 11.3 | 10.0 |
| ■ Casaba, fresh | 1/4 | 115 | 0.4 | 0.1 | 0.0 | 27.0 | 23.3 |
| ■ Cherimoya, fresh | 1 | 405 | 3.4 | n/a | 0.0 | 96.8 | n/a |
| Cherries, canned | | | | | | | |
| ■ Maraschino | 1 | 10 | 0.0 | 0.0 | 0.0 | 3.0 | 3.0 |
| ■ Sweet, water-packed | 1/2 cup | 57 | 0.2 | 0.0 | 0.0 | 14.6 | 12.7 |
| ■ Sweet, in heavy syrup | 1/2 cup | 105 | 0.2 | 0.0 | 0.0 | 26.9 | 25.0 |
| Cherries, fresh | | | | | | | |
| ■ Sour, red | 1/2 cup | 39 | 0.2 | 0.1 | 0.0 | 9.4 | 6.6 |
| ■ Sweet | 1/2 cup | 46 | 0.1 | 0.0 | 0.0 | 11.6 | 9.3 |
| Coconut, fresh, shredded | 2 tb. | 35 | 3.4 | 3.0 | 0.0 | 1.5 | 0.6 |
| Dried, flaked, sweetened | 2 tb. | 44 | 3.0 | 2.6 | n/a | 4.4 | 4.0 |
| ■ Crab apples, fresh | 1 | 25 | 0.1 | 0.0 | 0.0 | 6.6 | 0.6 |
| ■ Cranberries, fresh | 1/2 cup | 22 | 0.1 | 0.0 | 0.0 | 5.8 | 1.9 |
| ■ Dried | 1 oz. | 92 | 0.0 | 0.0 | 0.0 | 23.4 | 22.0 |
| ■ Sauce, jellied | 1/2 cup | 200 | 0.0 | 0.0 | 0.0 | 52.0 | 34.0 |
| ■ Currants, red, fresh | 1/2 cup | 31 | 0.1 | 0.0 | 0.0 | 7.7 | 4.1 |
| ■ Dates, domestic | 1 | 23 | 0.0 | 0.0 | 0.0 | 6.2 | 5.3 |
| ■ Elderberries, fresh | 1/2 cup | 53 | 0.4 | 0.0 | 0.0 | 13.3 | n/a |
| ■ Figs, fresh | 1 | 37 | 0.2 | 0.0 | 0.0 | 9.6 | 8.1 |
| ■ Canned, in light syrup | 1/2 cup | 87 | 0.1 | 0.0 | 0.0 | 22.6 | 20.4 |
| ■ Dried | 1 | 47 | 0.2 | 0.0 | 0.0 | 12.1 | 9.1 |

■ Contains less than 20% fat
n/a Not available

| Item | SERVING | CAL-ORIES | FAT GRAMS | SAT. FAT GRAMS | TRANS FAT GRAMS | CARB. GRAMS | SUGAR GRAMS |
|---|---|---|---|---|---|---|---|
| Fruit cocktail, canned | | | | | | | |
| ■ In heavy syrup | 1/2 cup | 90 | 0.0 | 0.0 | 0.0 | 23.0 | 22.0 |
| ■ In juice | 1/2 cup | 60 | 0.0 | 0.0 | 0.0 | 15.0 | 14.0 |
| Fruit salad, canned | | | | | | | |
| ■ In heavy syrup | 1/2 cup | 93 | 0.1 | 0.0 | 0.0 | 24.4 | 23.1 |
| ■ Water-packed | 1/2 cup | 37 | 0.1 | 0.0 | 0.0 | 9.6 | n/a |
| ■ Gooseberries, fresh | 1/2 cup | 33 | 0.4 | 0.0 | 0.0 | 7.6 | n/a |
| ■ In light syrup | 1/2 cup | 92 | 0.3 | 0.0 | 0.0 | 23.6 | n/a |
| ■ Grapefruit, fresh | 1 | 120 | 0.0 | 0.0 | 0.0 | 32.0 | 20.0 |
| ■ Canned in light syrup | 1/2 cup | 76 | 0.1 | 0.0 | 0.0 | 19.6 | 19.1 |
| ■ Canned in water | 1/2 cup | 44 | 0.1 | 0.0 | 0.0 | 11.2 | 10.7 |
| Grapes, fresh | | | | | | | |
| ■ Concord | 1/2 cup | 31 | 0.2 | 0.1 | 0.0 | 7.9 | 7.5 |
| ■ Emperor | 1/2 cup | 55 | 0.1 | 0.0 | 0.0 | 14.5 | 12.4 |
| ■ Thompson | 1/2 cup | 55 | 0.1 | 0.0 | 0.0 | 14.5 | 12.4 |
| ■ Guava, fresh | 1 | 25 | 0.4 | 0.1 | 0.0 | 5.3 | n/a |
| ■ Honeydew, fresh, cubed | 1/2 cup | 31 | 0.1 | 0.0 | 0.0 | 7.7 | 6.9 |
| ■ Kiwi, fresh | 1 | 46 | 0.4 | 0.0 | 0.0 | 11.1 | 6.8 |
| ■ Kumquat, fresh | 1 | 13 | 0.2 | 0.0 | 0.0 | 3.0 | 1.8 |
| ■ Leechees, fresh | 1 | 6 | 0.0 | 0.0 | 0.0 | 1.6 | 1.5 |
| ■ Lemons, fresh | 1 | 17 | 0.2 | 0.0 | 0.0 | 5.4 | 1.5 |
| ■ Lemon juice | 1 tb. | 4 | 0.0 | 0.0 | 0.0 | 1.3 | 0.4 |
| ■ Lemon peel/zest | 1 tsp. | 1 | 0.0 | 0.0 | 0.0 | 0.3 | 0.1 |
| ■ Limes, fresh | 1 | 20 | 0.0 | 0.0 | 0.0 | 7.0 | 0.0 |
| ■ Lime juice | 1 tb. | 4 | 0.0 | 0.0 | 0.0 | 1.3 | 0.3 |
| ■ Loganberries, fresh | 1/2 cup | 31 | 0.4 | 0.0 | 0.0 | 6.9 | 3.3 |
| ■ Loquats, fresh | 1 | 8 | 0.0 | 0.0 | 0.0 | 1.9 | n/a |
| ■ Mango, fresh | 1/2 | 67 | 0.3 | 0.1 | 0.0 | 17.6 | 15.3 |
| Mixed fruit | | | | | | | |
| ■ Canned, chunky, in juice | 1/2 cup | 60 | 0.0 | 0.0 | 0.0 | 15.0 | 14.0 |
| ■ Dried | 2 oz. | 138 | 0.3 | 0.0 | 0.0 | 36.3 | n/a |
| ■ Frozen, sweetened | 1/2 cup | 93 | 0.4 | 0.1 | 0.0 | 22.9 | 20.8 |
| ■ Mulberries, fresh | 1/2 cup | 30 | 0.3 | 0.0 | 0.0 | 6.9 | 5.7 |
| ■ Nectarines, fresh | 1 | 70 | 0.5 | 0.0 | 0.0 | 16.0 | 12.0 |
| ■ Oranges, fresh | 1 | 62 | 0.2 | 0.0 | 0.0 | 15.4 | 12.3 |
| ■ Mandarin, canned in juice | 1/2 cup | 46 | 0.0 | 0.0 | 0.0 | 11.9 | 11.0 |
| ■ Papaya, fresh | 1/2 | 59 | 0.2 | 0.1 | 0.0 | 14.9 | 9.0 |
| ■ Passion fruit, fresh | 1 | 17 | 0.1 | 0.0 | 0.0 | 4.2 | 2.0 |
| ■ Peaches, fresh | 1 | 38 | 0.2 | 0.0 | 0.0 | 9.4 | 7.9 |
| ■ Canned in light syrup | 1/2 cup | 68 | 0.0 | 0.0 | 0.0 | 18.3 | 16.6 |
| ■ Canned in water | 1/2 cup | 29 | 0.1 | 0.0 | 0.0 | 7.5 | 5.9 |
| ■ Dried | 1/2 cup | 191 | 0.6 | 0.1 | 0.0 | 49.1 | 33.4 |
| ■ Frozen, unsweetened | 1/2 cup | 118 | 0.2 | 0.0 | 0.0 | 30.0 | 27.7 |
| ■ Pears, fresh | 1 | 96 | 0.2 | 0.0 | 0.0 | 25.7 | 16.3 |
| ■ Asian | 1 | 116 | 0.6 | 0.0 | 0.0 | 29.3 | 19.4 |
| ■ Canned in juice | 1/2 cup | 80 | 0.0 | 0.0 | 0.0 | 21.0 | 17.0 |
| ■ Dried | 1/2 cup | 236 | 0.6 | 0.0 | 0.0 | 62.7 | 56.0 |

■ Contains less than 20% fat

57

n/a Not available

| Item | SERVING | CAL-ORIES | FAT GRAMS | SAT. FAT GRAMS | TRANS FAT GRAMS | CARB. GRAMS | SUGAR GRAMS |
|---|---|---|---|---|---|---|---|
| ■ Persimmon, fresh | 1 | 32 | 0.1 | n/a | 0.0 | 8.4 | n/a |
| ■ Pineapple, fresh, diced | 1/2 cup | 37 | 0.1 | 0.0 | 0.0 | 9.8 | 7.2 |
| ■ Canned, chunked, in juice | 1/2 cup | 70 | 0.0 | 0.0 | 0.0 | 17.0 | 15.0 |
| ■ Plantain, cooked, sliced | 1/2 cup | 89 | 0.1 | 0.1 | 0.0 | 24.0 | 10.8 |
| ■ Plums, fresh | 1 | 40 | 0.5 | n/a | 0.0 | 9.5 | 5.0 |
| ■ Canned in heavy syrup | 1/2 cup | 115 | 0.1 | 0.0 | 0.0 | 30.0 | 28.8 |
| ■ Pomegranate, fresh | 1 | 105 | 0.5 | 0.1 | 0.0 | 26.4 | 25.5 |
| ■ Prickly pears, fresh | 1 | 42 | 0.5 | 0.1 | 0.0 | 9.9 | n/a |
| Prunes | | | | | | | |
| ■ Cooked, no sugar | 1/2 cup | 158 | 0.3 | 0.0 | 0.0 | 41.6 | 23.9 |
| ■ Dried, uncooked | 1 | 20 | 0.0 | 0.0 | 0.0 | 5.4 | 3.2 |
| ■ Pummelo, fresh | 1/2 cup | 36 | 0.0 | n/a | 0.0 | 9.1 | n/a |
| ■ Quince, fresh | 1 | 52 | 0.1 | 0.0 | 0.0 | 14.1 | n/a |
| ■ Raisins, seedless | 1/2 cup | 260 | 0.0 | 0.0 | 0.0 | 62.0 | 58.0 |
| ■ Raspberries, fresh | 1/2 cup | 25 | 0.0 | 0.0 | 0.0 | 8.5 | n/a |
| ■ Frozen | 1/2 cup | 129 | 0.2 | 0.0 | 0.0 | 32.7 | 27.2 |
| ■ Rhubarb, cooked, w/sugar | 1/2 cup | 139 | 0.1 | 0.0 | 0.0 | 37.4 | 34.4 |
| ■ Sapodilla, fresh | 1 | 141 | 1.9 | 0.3 | 0.0 | 33.9 | n/a |
| ■ Starfruit, fresh | 1 | 28 | 0.3 | 0.0 | 0.0 | 6.1 | 3.6 |
| ■ Strawberries, fresh, sliced, cup | 1/2 cup | 27 | 0.3 | 0.0 | 0.0 | 6.4 | 3.9 |
| ■ Frozen | 1/2 cup | 122 | 0.2 | 0.0 | 0.0 | 33.1 | 30.6 |
| ■ Tamarind | 1 | 5 | 0.0 | 0.0 | 0.0 | 1.3 | 1.2 |
| ■ Tangerines, fresh | 1 | 45 | 0.3 | 0.0 | 0.0 | 11.2 | 8.9 |
| ■ Watermelon, fresh, diced | 1/2 cup | 23 | 0.1 | 0.0 | 0.0 | 5.7 | 4.7 |

## ICE CREAM, FROZEN YOGURT, & NONDAIRY FROZEN DESSERTS

**Ice Cream**
Chocolate

| Item | SERVING | CAL-ORIES | FAT GRAMS | SAT. FAT GRAMS | TRANS FAT GRAMS | CARB. GRAMS | SUGAR GRAMS |
|---|---|---|---|---|---|---|---|
| Baskin-Robbins | 1/2 cup | 216 | 14.0 | 9.0 | 0.0 | 33.0 | 31.0 |
| Baskin-Robbins, Chocolate Ribbon | 1/2 cup | 240 | 12.0 | 8.0 | 0.0 | 31.0 | 31.0 |
| Ben & Jerry's New York Super Fudge Chunk | 1/2 cup | 310 | 20.0 | 11.0 | 0.0 | 30.0 | 25.0 |
| Dreyer's | 1/2 cup | 150 | 8.0 | 4.5 | 0.0 | 17.0 | 15.0 |
| Dreyer's Slow Churned Light, Fudge Tracks | 1/2 cup | 120 | 4.0 | 2.5 | 0.0 | 18.0 | 13.0 |
| ■ Häagen-Dazs Chocolate Fudge Brownie, low fat | 1/2 cup | 190 | 2.5 | 1.5 | 0.0 | 34.0 | 20.0 |
| Coconut Ice Cream in natural shell, Trader Joe's | 1 | 156 | 7.0 | 6.0 | n/a | 22.0 | 21.0 |
| Coffee, Häagen-Dazs | 1/2 cup | 270 | 18.0 | 11.0 | 0.5 | 21.0 | 21.0 |
| Cookies n' Cream, Baskin-Robbins | 1/2 cup | 280 | 15.0 | 8.0 | n/a | 32.0 | 27.0 |
| Dreyer's | 1/2 cup | 160 | 70.0 | 4.5 | 0.0 | 19.0 | 14.0 |
| Drumstick, Nestlé Foods | 1 | 159 | 9.0 | 4.4 | 0.0 | 18.0 | n/a |

■ Contains less than 20% fat
n/a Not available

| Item | SERVING | CAL-ORIES | FAT GRAMS | SAT. FAT GRAMS | TRANS FAT GRAMS | CARB. GRAMS | SUGAR GRAMS |
|---|---|---|---|---|---|---|---|
| Dibs, Dreyers, Vanilla w/Nestlé Crunch Coating | 26 pieces | 380 | 28.0 | 20.0 | 0.0 | 29.0 | 24.0 |
| Eskimo Pie bar, w/dark chocolate | 1 | 160 | 10.0 | 8.0 | 0.0 | 15.0 | 11.0 |
| No added sugar, reduced fat | 1 | 120 | 8.0 | 6.0 | 0.0 | 13.0 | 4.0 |
| ■ Fudgesicle | 1 | 90 | 1.5 | 1.0 | 0.0 | 16.0 | 13.0 |
| ■ Fat free | 1 | 65 | 0.3 | 0.2 | 0.0 | 13.7 | 10.3 |
| ■ No sugar added | 1 | 44 | 0.4 | 0.2 | 0.0 | 9.4 | 1.7 |
| ■ Breyer's Heart Smart Fudge Bar | 1 | 100 | 1.5 | 1.0 | 0.0 | 21.0 | 15.0 |
| Half Baked, Ben & Jerry's | 1/2 cup | 280 | 14.0 | 9.0 | 0.0 | 34.0 | 26.0 |
| Half Baked Body & Soul | 1/2 cup | 190 | 8.0 | 5.0 | 0.0 | 29.0 | 19.0 |
| Klondike Bar, light, no sugar added | 1 | 170 | 9.0 | 8.0 | 0.0 | 21.0 | 7.0 |
| No sugar added | | | | | | | |
| Baskin-Robbins Mad About Chocolate | 1/2 cup | 160 | 4.0 | 3.0 | 0.0 | 35.0 | 6.0 |
| Dreyer's Strawberry | 1/2 cup | 90 | 3.0 | 1.5 | 0.0 | 13.0 | 4.0 |
| ■ Dreyer's Fat-free Vanilla-Raspberry Swirl | 1/2 cup | 90 | 0.0 | 0.0 | 0.0 | 19.0 | 4.0 |
| Sandwich | 1 | 144 | 5.6 | 3.2 | n/a | 21.8 | 14.8 |
| Strawberry, Häagen-Dazs | 1/2 cup | 250 | 16.0 | 10.0 | 0.5 | 23.0 | 22.0 |
| Vanilla | | | | | | | |
| Baskin-Robbins | 1/2 cup | 260 | 16.0 | 10.0 | 0.0 | 26.0 | 26.0 |
| Ben & Jerry's Organic | 1/2 oz. | 34 | 2.2 | 1.6 | n/a | 2.8 | 2.5 |
| Dreyer's Slow Churned Light, French Silk | 1/2 cup | 130 | 4.5 | 3.0 | n/a | 19.0 | 14.0 |
| Dreyer's Slow Churned Light, Vanilla | 1/2 cup | 100 | 3.5 | 2.0 | 0.0 | 15.0 | 11.0 |
| Soft serve | 1/2 cup | 140 | 4.5 | 3.0 | n/a | 22.0 | 19.0 |
| **Frozen Yogurt** | | | | | | | |
| ■ Baskin-Robbins Perils of Praline | 1/2 cup | 190 | 3.5 | 1.5 | n/a | 37.0 | 34.0 |
| ■ Ben & Jerry's Half Baked, low fat | 1/2 cup | 190 | 3.0 | 1.5 | 0.0 | 35.0 | 23.0 |
| ■ Cherry Garcia, low fat | 1/2 cup | 170 | 3.0 | 2.0 | 0.0 | 32.0 | 22.0 |
| ■ Chocolate Fudge Brownie, low fat | 1/2 cup | 190 | 2.5 | 1.5 | 0.0 | 36.0 | 23.0 |
| Nonfat | | | | | | | |
| Dreyer's Strawberry | 1/2 cup | 100 | 0.0 | 0.0 | 0.0 | 22.0 | 15.0 |
| ■ Dreyer's Vanilla Chocolate Swirl | 1/2 cup | 90 | 0.0 | 0.0 | 0.0 | 19.0 | 13.0 |
| **Nondairy Frozen Desserts** | | | | | | | |
| Mocha Mix, Mocha Almond Fudge | 1/2 cup | 140 | 4.5 | 1.0 | 0.0 | 22.0 | 15.0 |
| Rice Dream, Vanilla | 1/2 cup | 150 | 6.0 | 0.5 | n/a | 23.0 | 17.0 |
| Mint Chocolate Chip | 1/2 cup | 170 | 8.0 | 1.5 | n/a | 26.0 | 19.0 |

■ Contains less than 20% fat
n/a Not available

| Item | SERVING | CAL-ORIES | FAT GRAMS | SAT. FAT GRAMS | TRANS FAT GRAMS | CARB. GRAMS | SUGAR GRAMS |
|---|---|---|---|---|---|---|---|
| Soy Delicious, Chocolate Velvet | ½ cup | 130 | 4.0 | 0.0 | 0.0 | 23.0 | 13.0 |
| Tofutti, Chocolate Supreme | ½ cup | 180 | 11.0 | 2.0 | n/a | 18.0 | 8.0 |
| ■ Chocolate Fudge, low fat | ½ cup | 120 | 2.0 | 1.0 | n/a | 25.0 | 18.0 |
| Cutie Tofutti, Vanilla | 1 each | 120 | 5.0 | 1.0 | 0.0 | 11.0 | 9.0 |
| ■ Wholesoy, organic, Swiss Chocolate | ½ cup | 180 | 2.5 | 0.0 | 0.0 | 21.0 | 18.0 |

**Others**

| Item | SERVING | CAL-ORIES | FAT GRAMS | SAT. FAT GRAMS | TRANS FAT GRAMS | CARB. GRAMS | SUGAR GRAMS |
|---|---|---|---|---|---|---|---|
| ■ Chocolate Mousse Bar, Weight Watchers | 1 | 60 | 0.5 | 0.0 | 0.0 | 14.0 | 9.0 |
| Cone w/o ice cream | | | | | | | |
| ■ Sugar, old-fashioned, Keebler | 1 | 48 | 0.6 | 0.1 | 0.0 | 10.2 | 3.7 |
| ■ Wafer/cake type | 1 | 17 | 0.3 | 0.1 | 0.0 | 3.2 | 0.2 |
| Fruit Bars | | | | | | | |
| Dreyer's Whole Fruit | | | | | | | |
| Coconut | 1 | 120 | 3.0 | 2.5 | 0.0 | 21.0 | 16.0 |
| ■ Lime | 1 | 80 | 0.0 | 0.0 | 0.0 | 20.0 | 19.0 |
| ■ Orange and Cream | 1 | 80 | 1.5 | 0.5 | 0.0 | 16.0 | 15.0 |
| ■ Fat Free Fruit and Freeze | 1 | 60 | 0.0 | 0.0 | 0.0 | 15.0 | 11.0 |
| ■ Good Humor/Breyer's Strawberry fruit juice bar | 1 | 120 | 0.0 | 0.0 | 0.0 | 30.0 | 23.0 |
| ■ Ice Milk, chocolate | ½ cup | 95 | 2.1 | 1.3 | n/a | 16.9 | 16.4 |
| ■ Popsicle, Cherry | 1 | 45 | 0.0 | 0.0 | 0.0 | 11.0 | 11.0 |
| ■ Sugar Free | 1 | 15 | 0.0 | 0.0 | 0.0 | 4.0 | 2.0 |
| ■ Sherbet, Orange | ½ cup | 120 | 1.0 | 0.5 | 0.0 | 26.0 | 22.0 |
| Sorbet | | | | | | | |
| ■ Chocolate, Häagen-Dazs | ½ cup | 120 | 0.0 | 0.0 | 0.0 | 28.0 | 20.0 |
| ■ Lemon, in natural shell, Trader Joe's | 1 | 80 | 0.0 | 0.0 | 0.0 | 19.0 | 17.0 |
| ■ Lemon, nonfat, Häagen-Dazs | ½ cup | 110 | 0.0 | 0.0 | 0.0 | 28.0 | 27.5 |
| ■ Mango, Häagen-Dazs | ½ cup | 119 | 0.0 | 0.0 | 0.0 | 36.7 | 35.8 |
| ■ Orange, in natural shell, Trader Joe's | 1 | 89 | 0.0 | 0.0 | 0.0 | 22.0 | 21.0 |
| ■ Peach, nonfat, Häagen-Dazs | ½ cup | 130 | 0.0 | 0.0 | 0.0 | 33.0 | 29.0 |
| ■ Raspberry Sorbet & Vanilla Yogurt Bar, Häagen-Dazs | 1 | 90 | 0.0 | 0.0 | 0.0 | 21.0 | 15.0 |
| ■ Strawberry, nonfat, Häagen-Dazs | ½ cup | 120 | 0.0 | 0.0 | 0.0 | 30.0 | 29.5 |

## JAMS & JELLIES

| Item | SERVING | CAL-ORIES | FAT GRAMS | SAT. FAT GRAMS | TRANS FAT GRAMS | CARB. GRAMS | SUGAR GRAMS |
|---|---|---|---|---|---|---|---|
| ■ Apple Butter | 1 tb. | 31 | 0.0 | 0.0 | 0.0 | 7.7 | 6.4 |
| ■ Fruit spread, St. Dalfour's | 1 tb. | 60 | 0.1 | 0.0 | 0.0 | 14.6 | 14.6 |
| Lemon curd | 1 tb. | 60 | 6.0 | 3.0 | n/a | 4.0 | 4.0 |
| ■ Marmalade, orange | 1 tb. | 50 | 0.0 | 0.0 | 0.0 | 13.0 | 12.0 |
| ■ Simply Fruit 100% fruit spread | 1 tb. | 40 | 0.0 | 0.0 | 0.0 | 10.0 | 8.0 |
| ■ Strawberry preserves | 1 tb. | 50 | 0.0 | 0.0 | 0.0 | 13.0 | 12.0 |
| ■ Smucker's, sugar free | 1 tb. | 10 | 0.0 | 0.0 | 0.0 | 5.0 | 0.0 |

■ Contains less than 20% fat
n/a Not available

| Item | SERVING | CAL-ORIES | FAT GRAMS | SAT. FAT GRAMS | TRANS FAT GRAMS | CARB. GRAMS | SUGAR GRAMS |
|---|---|---|---|---|---|---|---|

## MEAT

**Beef**

| Item | SERVING | CAL-ORIES | FAT GRAMS | SAT. FAT GRAMS | TRANS FAT GRAMS | CARB. GRAMS | SUGAR GRAMS |
|---|---|---|---|---|---|---|---|
| Beefalo | 3 oz. | 160 | 5.4 | 2.3 | n/a | 0.0 | 0.0 |
| Brisket, flat lean, braised | 3 oz. | 185 | 8.6 | 3.1 | 0.7 | 0.0 | 0.0 |
| Chuck | | | | | | | |
| Arm, lean, braised | 3 oz. | 173 | 5.7 | 2.2 | 0.4 | 0.0 | 0.0 |
| Blade, lean, braised | 3 oz. | 215 | 11.3 | 4.4 | 0.4 | 0.0 | 0.0 |
| Ground | | | | | | | |
| Extra-lean, broiled, 10% fat | 3 oz. | 151 | 6.2 | 2.5 | 0.1 | 0.0 | 0.0 |
| Lean, broiled | 3 oz. | 213 | 13.2 | 5.0 | 0.6 | 0.0 | 0.0 |
| Rib eye, lean, broiled | 3 oz. | 174 | 7.7 | 2.9 | 1.5 | 0.0 | 0.0 |
| Round | | | | | | | |
| Bottom, lean, braised | 3 oz. | 173 | 6.5 | 2.2 | 0.2 | 0.0 | 0.0 |
| Eye, lean, roasted | 3 oz. | 138 | 3.5 | 1.2 | 0.0 | 0.0 | 0.0 |
| Tip, lean, roasted | 3 oz. | 148 | 5.3 | 1.9 | 0.2 | 0.0 | 0.0 |
| Top, lean, roasted | 3 oz. | 169 | 4.3 | 1.5 | n/a | 0.0 | 0.0 |
| Short ribs, lean, braised | 3 oz. | 251 | 15.4 | 6.6 | n/a | 0.0 | 0.0 |
| Sirloin, lean, broiled | 3 oz. | 155 | 5.4 | 2.1 | 0.6 | 0.0 | 0.0 |
| Steak, flank, lean, broiled | 3 oz. | 165 | 7.1 | 2.9 | 0.7 | 0.0 | 0.0 |
| Tenderloin, lean, broiled | 3 oz. | 164 | 6.7 | 2.6 | 0.5 | 0.0 | 0.0 |

**Game**

| Item | SERVING | CAL-ORIES | FAT GRAMS | SAT. FAT GRAMS | TRANS FAT GRAMS | CARB. GRAMS | SUGAR GRAMS |
|---|---|---|---|---|---|---|---|
| ■ Buffalo, roasted | 3 oz. | 111 | 1.5 | 0.5 | 0.0 | 0.0 | 0.0 |
| Rabbit, domestic, stewed | 3 oz. | 168 | 6.9 | 2.0 | 0.0 | 0.0 | 0.0 |
| ■ Rabbit, wild, stewed | 3 oz. | 147 | 3.0 | 0.9 | 0.0 | 0.0 | 0.0 |
| Venison, ground | 4.0 oz. | 130 | 3.0 | 1.5 | n/a | 0.0 | 1.0 |
| ■ Venison, roasted | 3 oz. | 134 | 2.7 | 1.1 | 0.0 | 0.0 | 0.0 |

**Ham**

| Item | SERVING | CAL-ORIES | FAT GRAMS | SAT. FAT GRAMS | TRANS FAT GRAMS | CARB. GRAMS | SUGAR GRAMS |
|---|---|---|---|---|---|---|---|
| Cured, lean | 3 oz. | 140 | 6.5 | 2.2 | 0.0 | 0.4 | 0.0 |
| Fresh, roasted, lean & fat | 3 oz. | 232 | 15.0 | 5.5 | 0.0 | 0.0 | 0.0 |
| Picnic, simmered, lean | 3 oz. | 142 | 7.2 | 2.4 | 0.0 | 0.4 | 0.0 |
| Cured, extra-lean | 3 oz. | 116 | 4.2 | 1.4 | 0.0 | 0.4 | n/a |

**Lamb**

| Item | SERVING | CAL-ORIES | FAT GRAMS | SAT. FAT GRAMS | TRANS FAT GRAMS | CARB. GRAMS | SUGAR GRAMS |
|---|---|---|---|---|---|---|---|
| Chop | | | | | | | |
| Loin, broiled, lean | 3 oz. | 184 | 8.3 | 3.0 | n/a | 0.0 | 0.0 |
| Loin, broiled, lean & fat | 3 oz. | 269 | 19.6 | 8.4 | n/a | 0.0 | 0.0 |
| Rib | | | | | | | |
| Broiled, lean | 3 oz. | 200 | 11.0 | 4.0 | n/a | 0.0 | 0.0 |
| Broiled, lean & fat | 3 oz. | 307 | 25.2 | 10.8 | n/a | 0.0 | 0.0 |
| Shoulder | | | | | | | |
| Broiled, lean | 3 oz. | 170 | 7.7 | 2.9 | n/a | 0.0 | 0.0 |
| Broiled, lean & fat | 3 oz. | 239 | 16.6 | 7.1 | n/a | 0.0 | 0.0 |
| Leg, lean, roasted | 3 oz. | 153 | 5.7 | 2.0 | n/a | 0.0 | 0.0 |

■ Contains less than 20% fat
n/a Not available

| Item | SERVING | CAL-ORIES | FAT GRAMS | SAT. FAT GRAMS | TRANS FAT GRAMS | CARB. GRAMS | SUGAR GRAMS |
|---|---|---|---|---|---|---|---|
| **Pork** | | | | | | | |
| Boston butt, roasted, lean | 3 oz. | 197 | 12.2 | 4.4 | n/a | 0.0 | 0.0 |
| Chitterlings, simmered | 3 oz. | 202 | 17.3 | 8.1 | 0.0 | 0.0 | 0.0 |
| Chop, broiled | | | | | | | |
| Loin | 3 oz. | 199 | 11.8 | 4.3 | 0.0 | 0.0 | 0.0 |
| Rib, lean & fat | 3 oz. | 221 | 13.4 | 4.9 | 0.0 | 0.0 | 0.0 |
| Loin, roasted | 3 oz. | 147 | 5.2 | 1.8 | 0.0 | 0.0 | 0.0 |
| Blade, lean | 3 oz. | 210 | 12.6 | 4.5 | 0.0 | 0.0 | 0.0 |
| Sirloin, lean | 3 oz. | 168 | 7.0 | 2.5 | 0.0 | 0.0 | 0.0 |
| Sirloin, lean & fat | 3 oz. | 176 | 8.0 | 2.9 | 0.0 | 0.0 | 0.0 |
| Spareribs, braised, lean & fat | 3 oz. | 338 | 25.8 | 9.5 | n/a | 0.0 | 0.0 |
| Tenderloin, roasted, lean | 3 oz. | 130 | 4.0 | 1.5 | 0.0 | 0.0 | 0.0 |
| **Prepared or Processed Meats** | | | | | | | |
| Bacon, regular, pan-fried | 3 pieces | 103 | 7.9 | 2.6 | 0.0 | 0.3 | 0.0 |
| Canadian, pan-fried | 2 pieces | 86 | 3.9 | 1.3 | 0.0 | 0.6 | 0.0 |
| Bacon, imitation | | | | | | | |
| Bits, Bacos | 1 oz. | 118 | 4.5 | n/a | 0.0 | 7.7 | n/a |
| Meatless, strips | 1 each | 16 | 1.5 | 0.2 | 0.0 | 0.3 | 0.0 |
| Turkey, Louis Rich | 2 oz. | 142 | 11.5 | 3.0 | 0.0 | 0.9 | 0.9 |
| Beef, corned | | | | | | | |
| Canned | 2 oz. | 120 | 7.0 | 3.0 | 0.0 | 0.0 | 0.0 |
| Cooked | 2 oz. | 142 | 10.6 | 3.6 | 0.0 | 0.2 | 0.0 |
| Beef, sliced, Buddig | 2 oz. | 78 | 3.6 | 1.4 | 0.0 | 0.4 | n/a |
| ■ Beef jerky | 1 oz. | 81 | 1.0 | 0.0 | 0.0 | 3.0 | 3.0 |
| Brockwurst, pork/veal | 2 oz. | 158 | 14.6 | 5.8 | 0.0 | 0.2 | 0.0 |
| Bologna | | | | | | | |
| Beef, Boar's Head | 1 slice | 59 | 6.4 | 2.0 | 0.0 | 0.0 | 0.0 |
| Beef & Pork | 1 slice | 87 | 7.0 | 2.6 | 0.0 | 1.6 | 1.3 |
| Chicken, Empire Kosher | 1 slice | 40 | 3.0 | 0.8 | 0.0 | 0.0 | 0.0 |
| Turkey, Empire Kosher | 1 slice | 40 | 2.0 | 1.0 | 0.0 | 0.3 | 0.0 |
| Turkey, Healthy Choice | 1 slice | 30 | 1.0 | 0.5 | 0.0 | 3.0 | 1.0 |
| Turkey, Louis Rich | 1 slice | 52 | 3.7 | 1.1 | 0.0 | 1.4 | 0.3 |
| Bratwurst, pork | 1 each | 281 | 24.8 | 8.6 | 0.0 | 2.1 | 0.0 |
| Braunschweiger, pork | 2 oz. | 185 | 16.2 | 5.3 | 0.0 | 1.8 | 0.0 |
| ■ Chicken breast, oven-roasted, Healthy Choice | 1 slice | 25 | 0.0 | 0.0 | 0.0 | 2.0 | 1.0 |
| Chorizo, pork & beef | 1 each | 273 | 23.0 | 8.6 | n/a | 1.1 | 0.0 |
| Corn dog, beef | 1 each | 210 | 10.0 | 4.0 | 0.5 | 24 | 6.0 |
| Frankfurter/hot dog | | | | | | | |
| Beef, Boar's Head, natural casing | 1 each | 120 | 10.0 | 4.0 | 0.0 | 2.0 | 0.0 |
| Beef, Hebrew National 97% fat free | 1 each | 45 | 1.5 | 1.0 | 1.0 | 3.0 | 0.0 |
| Beef, Oscar Meyer | 1 each | 147 | 13.6 | 5.6 | 1.0 | 1.1 | 0.7 |
| ■ Beef, Oscar Meyer Fat Free | 1 each | 37 | 0.3 | 0.1 | 0.0 | 2.2 | 1.1 |
| Chicken, Beef, & Pork, Hoffy | 1 each | 90 | 6.0 | 2.0 | 0.0 | 4.0 | 1.0 |

■ Contains less than 20% fat
n/a Not available

| Item | SERVING | CAL-ORIES | FAT GRAMS | SAT. FAT GRAMS | TRANS FAT GRAMS | CARB. GRAMS | SUGAR GRAMS |
|---|---|---|---|---|---|---|---|
| Chicken franks | 1 each | 116 | 8.8 | 2.5 | 0.0 | 3.1 | 0.0 |
| Low-fat, Healthy Choice | 1 each | 80 | 2.5 | 1.0 | 0.0 | 7.0 | 2.0 |
| Hot dog, turkey, Applegate Farms | 1 each | 80 | 6.0 | 2.0 | 0.0 | 0.0 | 0.0 |
| Turkey, Empire Kosher | 1 each | 90 | 6.0 | 1.5 | 0.0 | 0.0 | 0.0 |
| Turkey, Shelton, uncured, smoked | 1 each | 150 | 11.0 | 3.5 | n/a | 2.0 | n/a |
| ■ Veggie Dogs, Yves | 1 each | 50 | 0.0 | 0.0 | 0.0 | 1.0 | 0.0 |
| Ham, chopped, canned | 1 oz. | 68 | 5.3 | 1.8 | n/a | 0.1 | 0.0 |
| Ham, sliced, Buddig | 1 oz. | 46 | 2.6 | 0.9 | 0.0 | 0.3 | n/a |
| Brown sugar-baked, lean slices | 1 oz. | 34 | 0.7 | 0.2 | 0.0 | 1.5 | 1.0 |
| Low-fat, Oscar Meyer | 1 oz. | 31 | 0.9 | 0.4 | 0.0 | 0.8 | 0.5 |
| Ham, deviled spread | 2 oz. | 150 | 12.0 | 3.5 | 0.0 | 0.0 | 0.0 |
| Ham, turkey | 1 oz. | 32 | 1.2 | 0.5 | 0.0 | 0.2 | 0.2 |
| Headcheese, Oscar Meyer | 1 oz. | 52 | 3.8 | 1.2 | n/a | 0.0 | 0.0 |
| Kielbasa, pork & beef | 1 each | 81 | 7.0 | 2.6 | 0.0 | 0.6 | 0.0 |
| Kielbasa, turkey, Louis Rich | 1 each | 41 | 2.3 | 0.7 | 0.0 | 0.7 | 0.5 |
| ■ Kielbasa, turkey/pork/beef, Healthy Choice | 1 each | 35 | 0.8 | 0.3 | 0.0 | 3.0 | 1.5 |
| Knockwurst | 1 each | 209 | 18.8 | 6.9 | 1.0 | 2.2 | 0.0 |
| Liverwurst | 2 oz. | 190 | 17.0 | 6.0 | 0.0 | 2.0 | 0.0 |
| Mortadella, beef & pork | 1 oz. | 88 | 7.2 | 2.7 | n/a | 0.9 | 0.0 |
| Olive loaf, Boar's Head | 1 oz. | 64 | 5.9 | 2.2 | n/a | 0.0 | 0.0 |
| Pancetta | 1 oz. | 155 | 7.7 | 3.9 | 0.0 | 0.0 | 0.0 |
| Pastrami | | | | | | | |
| Beef | 2 oz. | 60 | 1.0 | 0.5 | 0.0 | 0.0 | 0.0 |
| Sliced, Buddig | 1 oz. | 40 | 1.8 | 0.9 | 0.0 | 0.3 | n/a |
| Turkey | 1 oz. | 35 | 1.3 | 0.5 | 0.0 | 0.0 | 0.0 |
| Turkey, Empire Kosher | 3 slices | 60 | 3.0 | 0.5 | 0.5 | 0.0 | 0.0 |
| Pâté | | | | | | | |
| Chicken liver, canned | 1 oz. | 57 | 3.7 | 1.1 | n/a | 1.9 | 0.0 |
| Goose liver, smoked, canned | 1 oz. | 131 | 12.4 | 4.1 | n/a | 1.3 | n/a |
| Pork liver | 1 oz. | 42 | 3.5 | 1.2 | 0.0 | 0.8 | 0.2 |
| Pepperoni, pork & beef | 1 oz. | 132 | 11.4 | 4.6 | n/a | 1.2 | 0.2 |
| Pig's feet, pickled | 3 oz. | 173 | 13.7 | 4.7 | 0.0 | 0.0 | 0.0 |
| Pork, salt, raw | 1 oz. | 212 | 22.8 | 8.3 | 0.0 | 0.0 | 0.0 |
| Potted meat, Libby's | 1 oz. | 57 | 4.0 | 1.0 | n/a | 0.0 | 0.0 |
| Salami | | | | | | | |
| Beef, lean, Hebrew National | 1 oz. | 45 | 2.5 | 1.5 | 0.0 | 0.0 | 0.0 |
| Beef | 1 slice | 75 | 6.5 | 3.0 | n/a | 0.0 | 0.0 |
| Pork | 1 slice | 115 | 9.6 | 3.4 | 0.0 | 0.5 | n/a |
| Turkey | 1 slice | 43 | 2.7 | 0.8 | 0.0 | 0.1 | 0.1 |
| Turkey, Empire Kosher | 1 slice | 40 | 2.0 | 0.7 | 0.0 | 0.0 | 0.0 |
| Sausage | | | | | | | |
| Beef | 2 oz. | 190 | 17.0 | 8.0 | 1.0 | 1.0 | 1.0 |
| Brown & Serve, Jones | 2 pieces | 190 | 18.0 | 6.0 | 0.0 | 1.0 | 0.0 |

■ Contains less than 20% fat

63

n/a Not available

| Item | SERVING | CAL-ORIES | FAT GRAMS | SAT. FAT GRAMS | TRANS FAT GRAMS | CARB. GRAMS | SUGAR GRAMS |
|---|---|---|---|---|---|---|---|
| Italian, turkey | 1 piece | 150 | 10.0 | 2.5 | 0.0 | 3.0 | 1.0 |
| Polish, pork | 2 oz. | 170 | 16.0 | 6.0 | 0.0 | 1.0 | 0.0 |
| Pork | 1 oz. | 76 | 5.7 | 1.6 | 0.0 | 0.0 | 0.0 |
| Link | 1 piece | 134 | 11.6 | 4.9 | 0.0 | 1.0 | n/a |
| Patty | 1 piece | 200 | 19.0 | 17.0 | 0.0 | 2.0 | 1.0 |
| Turkey, link | 1 piece | 46 | 2.8 | 0.8 | 0.0 | 1.0 | 0.0 |
| Vienna, Libby's | 1 piece | 50 | 4.7 | 0.8 | 0.0 | 0.0 | 0.0 |
| Scrapple, pork | 1 oz. | 60 | 4.1 | 1.5 | n/a | 4.1 | 0.0 |
| Spam, Hormel, original | 1 oz. | 88 | 7.7 | 2.8 | 0.0 | 0.9 | n/a |
| Lite | 1 oz. | 54 | 3.9 | 1.3 | 0.0 | 0.4 | 0.4 |
| ■ Turkey Breast, Boar's Head | 1 oz. | 41 | 0.3 | 0.0 | 0.0 | 0.0 | 0.0 |
| **Variety Meats, Beef** | | | | | | | |
| Brains | 3 oz. | 123 | 9.0 | 2.6 | 0.4 | 0.0 | 0.0 |
| Heart | 3 oz. | 140 | 4.0 | 1.2 | 0.1 | 0.1 | 0.0 |
| Kidney | 3 oz. | 134 | 4.0 | 0.9 | 0.2 | 0.0 | 0.0 |
| Liver | 3 oz. | 149 | 4.0 | 1.3 | 0.2 | 4.4 | 0.0 |
| Oxtail | 3 oz. | 207 | 11.4 | 4.8 | n/a | 0.0 | 0.0 |
| Sweetbreads | 3 oz. | 199 | 12.9 | 5.8 | n/a | 0.0 | 0.0 |
| Thymus | 3 oz. | 106 | 2.6 | 0.8 | 0.2 | 0.0 | 0.0 |
| Tongue | 3 oz. | 242 | 19.0 | 6.9 | 0.7 | 0.0 | 0.0 |
| Tripe | 3 oz. | 80 | 3.4 | 1.2 | 0.2 | 1.7 | 0.0 |
| **Veal** | | | | | | | |
| Breast, cooked | 3 oz. | 443 | 45.4 | 18.2 | n/a | 0.0 | 0.0 |
| Chop, braised | 3 oz. | 213 | 10.7 | 4.2 | n/a | 0.0 | 0.0 |
| Cubed, for stew, braised, lean | 3 oz. | 160 | 3.7 | 1.1 | n/a | 0.0 | 0.0 |
| Cutlet, braised | 3 oz. | 242 | 14.6 | 5.7 | n/a | 0.0 | 0.0 |
| Leg, roasted | | | | | | | |
| Lean | 3 oz. | 128 | 2.9 | 1.0 | n/a | 0.0 | 0.0 |
| Lean & fat | 3 oz. | 136 | 4.0 | 1.6 | n/a | 0.0 | 0.0 |
| Loin, roasted | | | | | | | |
| Lean | 3 oz. | 149 | 5.9 | 2.2 | n/a | 0.0 | 0.0 |
| Lean & fat | 3 oz. | 185 | 10.5 | 4.5 | n/a | 0.0 | 0.0 |
| Rib, roasted | | | | | | | |
| Lean | 3 oz. | 151 | 6.3 | 1.8 | n/a | 0.0 | 0.0 |
| Lean & fat | 3 oz. | 194 | 11.9 | 4.6 | n/a | 0.0 | 0.0 |
| Shoulder, roasted | | | | | | | |
| Lean | 3 oz. | 145 | 5.6 | 2.1 | n/a | 0.0 | 0.0 |
| Lean & fat | 3 oz. | 156 | 7.2 | 2.9 | n/a | 0.0 | 0.0 |
| Sirloin, roasted | | | | | | | |
| Lean | 3 oz. | 143 | 5.3 | 2.1 | n/a | 0.0 | 0.0 |
| Lean & fat | 3 oz. | 172 | 8.9 | 3.8 | n/a | 0.0 | 0.0 |
| **Miscellaneous** | | | | | | | |
| ■ Snails, steamed | 1 each | 14 | 0.0 | 0.0 | 0.0 | 0.8 | 0.4 |

■ Contains less than 20% fat
n/a Not available

| Item | SERVING | CAL-ORIES | FAT GRAMS | SAT. FAT GRAMS | TRANS FAT GRAMS | CARB. GRAMS | SUGAR GRAMS |
|---|---|---|---|---|---|---|---|

## NUTS, SEEDS, & NUT BUTTERS

| Item | SERVING | CAL-ORIES | FAT GRAMS | SAT. FAT GRAMS | TRANS FAT GRAMS | CARB. GRAMS | SUGAR GRAMS |
|---|---|---|---|---|---|---|---|
| Almond butter | 2 tb. | 203 | 18.9 | 1.8 | 0.0 | 6.8 | n/a |
| Almonds (1 oz. = 22) | 1 oz. | 164 | 14.4 | 1.1 | 0.0 | 5.6 | 1.4 |
| Beechnuts | 1 oz. | 163 | 14.2 | 1.6 | 0.0 | 9.5 | n/a |
| Brazil nuts (1 oz. = 6) | 1 oz. | 195 | 19.3 | 7.7 | 0.0 | 3.1 | 0.5 |
| Cashew butter | 2 tb. | 188 | 15.8 | 3.1 | 0.0 | 8.8 | n/a |
| Cashews (1 oz. = 18) | 1 oz. | 163 | 13.1 | 2.6 | 0.0 | 9.3 | 1.4 |
| ■ Chestnuts | 1 oz. | 64 | 0.3 | 0.1 | 0.0 | 13.9 | n/a |
| Coconut (see Fruits) | | | | | | | |
| Hazelnuts/filberts (1 oz. = 20) | 1 oz. | 178 | 17.2 | 1.3 | 0.0 | 4.7 | 1.2 |
| Macadamia nuts (1 oz. = 11) | 1 oz. | 204 | 21.6 | 3.4 | 0.0 | 3.8 | 1.2 |
| Mixed nuts | | | | | | | |
|   Oil-roasted, no peanuts | 1 oz. | 174 | 15.9 | 2.6 | 0.0 | 6.3 | 1.0 |
|   Dry-roasted w/peanuts | 1 oz. | 168 | 14.6 | 2.0 | 0.0 | 7.2 | n/a |
| Peanuts (1 oz. = 28) | | | | | | | |
|   Dry roasted | 1 oz. | 166 | 14.1 | 2.0 | 0.0 | 6.1 | 1.2 |
|   Honey roasted | 1 oz. | 180 | 13.0 | 2.5 | 0.0 | 9.0 | 7.0 |
|   Raw | 1 oz. | 161 | 14.0 | 1.9 | 0.0 | 4.6 | 1.1 |
| Peanut butter | | | | | | | |
|   Chunky | 2 tb. | 188 | 16.0 | 2.6 | 0.0 | 6.9 | 2.7 |
|   Low-fat, Jif | 2 tb. | 200 | 12.0 | 2.0 | 0.0 | 12.0 | 2.0 |
|   Smooth | 2 tb. | 188 | 16.1 | 3.3 | 0.0 | 6.3 | 3.0 |
| Pecans (1 oz. = 20 halves) | 1 oz. | 196 | 20.4 | 1.8 | 0.0 | 3.9 | 1.1 |
| Pine/pignolia nuts | 1 oz. | 191 | 19.4 | 1.4 | 0.0 | 3.7 | 1.0 |
| Pistachios (1 oz. = 47) | 1 oz. | 162 | 13.0 | 1.6 | 0.0 | 7.8 | 2.2 |
| Poppy seeds | 1 oz. | 151 | 12.7 | 1.4 | 0.0 | 6.7 | 3.9 |
| Pumpkin seeds | 1 oz. | 153 | 13.0 | 2.5 | 0.0 | 5.1 | 0.3 |
| Sesame seeds | 1 oz. | 162 | 14.1 | 2.0 | 0.0 | 6.7 | 0.1 |
| Sunflower seeds | 1 oz. | 162 | 14.1 | 1.5 | 0.0 | 5.3 | 0.7 |
| Tahini/sesame butter | 2 tb. | 178 | 15.9 | 2.2 | 0.0 | 6.5 | n/a |
| Trail mix, no coconut | 1 oz. | 131 | 8.3 | 1.6 | 0.0 | 12.7 | n/a |
| Walnuts (1 oz. = 14 halves) | | | | | | | |
|   Black | 1 oz. | 175 | 16.7 | 1.0 | 0.0 | 2.8 | 0.3 |
|   English | 1 oz. | 185 | 18.5 | 1.7 | 0.0 | 3.9 | 0.7 |

## PASTA & NOODLES

| Item | SERVING | CAL-ORIES | FAT GRAMS | SAT. FAT GRAMS | TRANS FAT GRAMS | CARB. GRAMS | SUGAR GRAMS |
|---|---|---|---|---|---|---|---|
| ■ Egg Barley (toasted farfel), Osem | 2 oz. | 190 | 0.5 | 0.0 | 0.0 | 40.0 | 1.0 |
| ■ Egg roll wrapper | 1 | 65 | 0.3 | 0.0 | 0.0 | 14.0 | 0.5 |
| ■ Gnocchi, Potato, Mediterranean | 1 cup | 250 | 1.0 | 0.0 | 0.0 | 56.0 | 2.0 |
| ■ Macaroni noodles, cooked | 1 cup | 197 | 0.9 | 0.1 | 0.0 | 39.7 | 0.9 |
| ■   Cooked al dente | 1 cup | 155 | 0.6 | n/a | 0.0 | n/a | n/a |
| ■   Spiral noodles, cooked | 1 cup | 189 | 0.9 | 0.1 | 0.0 | 38.0 | 0.9 |
| ■   Whole wheat, cooked | 1 cup | 174 | 0.8 | 0.1 | 0.0 | 37.2 | 1.1 |
| ■     Bionaturae, fusilli, dry | 2 oz. | 190 | 0.0 | 0.0 | 0.0 | 42.0 | 0.0 |

■ Contains less than 20% fat
n/a Not available

| Item | SERVING | CAL-ORIES | FAT GRAMS | SAT. FAT GRAMS | TRANS FAT GRAMS | CARB. GRAMS | SUGAR GRAMS |
|---|---|---|---|---|---|---|---|
| Noodles, chow mein, canned La Choy | ½ cup | 130 | 5.0 | 1.5 | 1.5 | 19.0 | 0.0 |
| ■ Egg, cooked | 1 cup | 213 | 2.4 | 0.5 | 0.0 | 39.7 | 0.5 |
| ■ Lasagna, dry | 2 oz. | 206 | 0.8 | 0.2 | 0.0 | 42.2 | 2.4 |
| ■ Rice cooked | 1 cup | 192 | 0.4 | 0.0 | 0.0 | 43.8 | 0.0 |
| ■ w/o egg, fettuccini | 1 cup | 197 | 0.9 | 0.0 | 0.0 | n/a | n/a |
| ■ w/o yolk, dry, Manischewitz | 2 oz. | 210 | 1.0 | 0.0 | 0.0 | 40.0 | 2.0 |
| ■ Pasta, fresh, refrigerated, Pasta Roni | 3 oz. | 245 | 2.0 | 0.3 | 0.0 | 46.6 | n/a |
| ■ Angel Hair Pasta w/herbs | 2 oz. | 320 | 3.0 | 0.5 | 0.0 | 39.0 | 3.0 |
| ■ Parmesano | 2.5 oz. | 400 | 4.0 | 1.5 | 0.0 | 46.0 | 3.0 |
| ■ Soba noodles, cooked | 1 cup | 113 | 0.1 | 0.0 | 0.0 | 24.4 | 0.0 |
| ■ Spaetzle, dry | ¼ cup | 180 | 1.5 | 0.0 | 0.0 | 33.0 | 2.0 |
| ■ Spaghetti, cooked | 1 cup | 197 | 0.9 | 0.1 | 0.0 | 39.7 | 0.9 |
| ■ Cooked al dente | 1 cup | 155 | 0.6 | n/a | 0.0 | n/a | n/a |
| ■ Whole wheat, cooked | 1 cup | 174 | 0.8 | 0.1 | 0.0 | 37.2 | 1.1 |
| ■ Udon noodles, Japanese, dry | 2 oz. | 206 | 1.6 | 0.0 | 0.0 | 39.2 | 1.0 |
| ■ Wonton wrapper | 3.5" square | 23 | 0.1 | 0.0 | 0.0 | 4.6 | n/a |

## POULTRY

The amount of trans fat in all *fried* poultry depends on the *cooking fat* used.

**Chicken**

| Item | SERVING | CAL-ORIES | FAT GRAMS | SAT. FAT GRAMS | TRANS FAT GRAMS | CARB. GRAMS | SUGAR GRAMS |
|---|---|---|---|---|---|---|---|
| Breast, baked or broiled | | | | | | | |
| No skin | 3.5 oz. | 164 | 3.5 | 1.0 | 0.0 | 0.0 | 0.0 |
| With skin | 3.5 oz. | 195 | 7.7 | 2.2 | 0.1 | 0.0 | 0.0 |
| Breast, fried | | | | | | | |
| No skin | 3.5 oz. | 186 | 4.7 | 1.3 | n/a | 0.5 | 0.0 |
| With skin | 3.5 oz. | 220 | 8.8 | 2.4 | n/a | 1.6 | n/a |
| Capon, with skin, roasted | 3.5 oz. | 227 | 11.6 | 3.2 | 0.1 | 0.0 | 0.0 |
| Fryer, leg, roasted | | | | | | | |
| Fried w/skin | 1 | 284 | 16.2 | 4.4 | n/a | 2.8 | n/a |
| No skin | 1 | 181 | 8.0 | 2.2 | 0.1 | 0.0 | 0.0 |
| With skin | 1 | 264 | 15.3 | 4.2 | 0.1 | 0.0 | 0.0 |
| Fryer, thigh, roasted | | | | | | | |
| Fried, w/skin | 1 | 238 | 14.2 | 3.8 | n/a | 7.8 | n/a |
| No skin | 1 | 109 | 5.7 | 1.6 | 0.2 | 0.0 | 0.0 |
| With skin | 1 | 153 | 9.6 | 2.7 | 0.2 | 0.0 | 0.0 |
| Fryer, wing, w/skin | | | | | | | |
| Fried | 1 | 159 | 10.7 | 2.9 | n/a | 5.4 | n/a |
| Roasted | 1 | 99 | 6.6 | 1.9 | 0.1 | 0.0 | 0.0 |
| Giblets, simmered | 3.5 oz. | 157 | 4.5 | 1.3 | 0.1 | 0.4 | 0.0 |
| Liver, simmered | 3.5 oz. | 166 | 6.5 | 2.0 | 0.1 | 0.9 | 0.0 |

**Game**

| Item | SERVING | CAL-ORIES | FAT GRAMS | SAT. FAT GRAMS | TRANS FAT GRAMS | CARB. GRAMS | SUGAR GRAMS |
|---|---|---|---|---|---|---|---|
| Buffalo, patties | 4.0 oz. | 330 | 22.0 | 11.0 | n/a | 0.0 | 0.0 |

■ Contains less than 20% fat
n/a Not available

| Item | SERVING | CAL-ORIES | FAT GRAMS | SAT. FAT GRAMS | TRANS FAT GRAMS | CARB. GRAMS | SUGAR GRAMS |
|---|---|---|---|---|---|---|---|
| **Duck** | | | | | | | |
| Breast, no skin, wild, raw | 3.5 oz. | 122 | 4.2 | 1.3 | n/a | 0.0 | 0.0 |
| Whole, no skin, domesticated, roasted | 3.5 oz. | 199 | 11.1 | 4.1 | n/a | 0.0 | 0.0 |
| With skin | 3.5 oz. | 334 | 28.1 | 9.6 | n/a | 0.0 | 0.0 |
| Cornish Game Hen, roasted | 4 oz. | 305 | 8.6 | 4.0 | n/a | 0.0 | n/a |
| **Goose, roasted** | | | | | | | |
| No skin | 3.5 oz. | 236 | 12.6 | 4.5 | n/a | 0.0 | 0.0 |
| With skin | 3.5 oz. | 303 | 21.8 | 6.8 | n/a | 0.0 | 0.0 |
| Liver, raw | 1 oz. | 38 | 1.2 | 0.5 | n/a | 1.8 | n/a |
| Guinea hen, roasted | 3.5 oz. | 258 | 18.1 | 5.0 | n/a | 0.0 | 0.0 |
| Pheasant, cooked | 3.5 oz. | 245 | 12.0 | 3.5 | n/a | 0.0 | 0.0 |
| Quail, cooked | 3.5 oz. | 232 | 14.0 | 3.9 | n/a | 0.0 | 0.0 |
| Squab, raw | 3.5 oz. | 292 | 23.6 | 8.4 | n/a | 0.0 | 0.0 |
| **Ostrich** | | | | | | | |
| Ground, broiled | 3.5 oz. | 174 | 7.0 | 1.8 | 0.2 | 0.0 | 0.0 |
| Steak, cooked | 3.5 oz. | 132 | 3.7 | 0.0 | 0.25 | 0.0 | 0.0 |
| **Turkey** | | | | | | | |
| **Breast, roasted** | | | | | | | |
| ■ No skin | 3.5 oz. | 134 | 0.7 | 0.2 | 0.0 | 0.0 | 0.0 |
| ■ With skin | 3.5 oz. | 152 | 3.2 | 0.9 | 0.0 | 0.0 | 0.0 |
| **Dark meat, roasted** | | | | | | | |
| No skin | 3.5 oz. | 186 | 7.2 | 2.4 | 0.0 | 0.0 | 0.0 |
| With skin | 3.5 oz. | 219 | 11.5 | 3.5 | 0.0 | 0.0 | 0.0 |
| Leg w/skin, roasted | 1 each | 417 | 13.3 | 4.1 | 0.0 | 0.0 | 0.0 |
| **Light meat, roasted** | | | | | | | |
| ■ No skin | 3.5 oz. | 156 | 3.2 | 1.0 | 0.0 | 0.0 | 0.0 |
| With skin | 3.5 oz. | 195 | 8.3 | 2.3 | 0.0 | 0.0 | 0.0 |
| **Lunchmeat, breast only** | | | | | | | |
| ■ Hickory-smoked fat-free, Louis Rich | 2.5 oz. | 58 | 0.5 | 0.2 | 0.0 | 2.5 | 0.8 |
| ■ Honey roasted, fat free | 2.5 oz. | 72 | 0.6 | 0.2 | 0.0 | 3.2 | 2.8 |
| Honey roasted, smoked, Healthy Choice | 2.5 oz. | 89 | 2.5 | 1.3 | 0.0 | 5.1 | 2.5 |
| ■ Oven roasted, Sara Lee | 2.5 oz. | 71 | 0.8 | 0.0 | 0.0 | 3.2 | 0.0 |
| ■ Oven roasted, fat free, Oscar Meyer | 2.5 oz. | 61 | 0.5 | 0.2 | 0.0 | 3.3 | 1.3 |
| Patty, from ground | 3.5 oz. | 233 | 13.1 | 3.4 | 0.2 | 0.0 | 0.0 |
| Sausage link | 1 each | 47 | 2.9 | 0.8 | 0.2 | 0.0 | 0.0 |
| Wing w/skin | 1 each | 426 | 23.1 | 6.3 | n/a | 0.0 | 0.0 |
| **PREPARED FOODS** | | | | | | | |
| Beans & franks, canned | 1 cup | 368 | 17.0 | 6.1 | n/a | 39.9 | 16.9 |
| Beef stew, homemade, w/vegetables | 1 cup | 230 | 8.0 | 1.5 | n/a | 28.0 | 5.0 |

■ Contains less than 20% fat
n/a Not available

* See note, page xli

| Item | SERVING | CAL-ORIES | FAT GRAMS | SAT. FAT GRAMS | TRANS FAT GRAMS | CARB. GRAMS | SUGAR GRAMS |
|---|---|---|---|---|---|---|---|
| Dinty Moore | 1 cup | 222 | 13.1 | 5.6 | n/a | 16.1 | 2.3 |
| ■ Beef stir fry w/vegetables, homemade | 8 oz. | 243 | 2.8 | n/a | n/a | 39.6 | n/a |
| Cheese fondue, homemade | 1 cup | 492 | 29.0 | 18.8 | n/a | 8.1 | n/a |
| Chicken & egg noodles, homemade | 1 serv. | 370 | 21.0 | 9.0 | n/a | 31.0 | 4.0 |
| Chicken fried steak, w/gravy | 1 serv. | 650 | 37.0 | 13.0 | n/a | 50.0 | 9.0 |
| Chicken, Noodle Rings, Hormel, microcup | 1 | 140 | 4.0 | 1.5 | 0.0 | 18.0 | 2.0 |
| Chicken stew, canned | 1 cup | 250 | 10.0 | 2.0 | n/a | 26.0 | 5.0 |
| Chicken stir-fry, w/almonds | 8 oz. | 262 | 13.6 | 1.8 | n/a | 15.4 | 3.2 |
| Chili | | | | | | | |
| ■    Black bean, mild, vegetarian, fat free, Health Valley | 1 cup | 160 | 1.0 | 0.0 | 0.0 | 28.0 | 7.0 |
| ■    Regular, Hormel | 1 cup | 240 | 4.4 | 1.8 | 0.0 | 33.7 | 4.6 |
| ■    Turkey | 1 cup | 203 | 2.8 | 0.7 | 0.0 | 25.6 | 5.7 |
| ■        Chunky Turkey Chili | 1.25 cup | 216 | 3.8 | 0.6 | 0.0 | n/a | n/a |
| ■    Vegetarian, Hormel | 1 cup | 205 | 0.7 | 0.1 | 0.0 | 38.0 | 6.2 |
| Chop suey, beef, no noodles | 1 cup | 271 | 15.1 | 3.7 | n/a | 12.4 | n/a |
| Chow mein, beef, no noodles | 6 oz. | 210 | 11.7 | 2.9 | n/a | 9.6 | n/a |
| Chow mein, chicken, no noodles | 6 oz. | 149 | 6.5 | 1.4 | n/a | 7.6 | n/a |
| Coq au vin | 1 serv. | 800 | 30.0 | 16.0 | n/a | n/a | n/a |
| Dinosaurs | 1 cup | 260 | 7.0 | 3.0 | n/a | 40.0 | 0.0 |
| Falafel, homemade | 2.5" patty | 57 | 3.0 | 0.4 | n/a | 5.4 | n/a |
| Hamburger Helper, beef w/macaroni & cheese | 1 cup | 340 | 15.1 | 7.7 | n/a | 21.8 | n/a |
| Hash, corned beef, Hormel | 1 cup | 390 | 24.0 | 11.0 | 1.0 | 22.0 | 1.0 |
| Hash, turkey | 1 cup | 212 | 8.4 | 2.0 | n/a | 15.6 | n/a |
| Lasagna, w/meat & sauce, homemade | 6 oz. | 216 | 8.1 | 3.8 | n/a | 21.9 | n/a |
| Macaroni & cheese, homemade | 1 cup | 260 | 7.0 | 2.4 | n/a | 38.9 | 7.9 |
| ■    Annie's, whole wheat shells & cheddar | 1 cup | 360 | 5.0 | 3.0 | 0.0 | 46.0 | 2.0 |
| Hormel, microcup, cheezy | 1 | 270 | 11.0 | 6.0 | 0.0 | 32.0 | 3.0 |
| Kraft, original, from mix | 1 cup | 220 | 4.0 | 2.5 | 0.0 | 39.0 | 6.0 |
| Cheesy alfredo, from mix | 1 cup | 410 | 19.0 | 5.0 | n/a | 49.0 | 8.0 |
| ■        Light, from mix | 1 cup | 290 | 4.5 | 2.5 | n/a | 48.0 | 7.0 |
| Thick 'n creamy, from mix | 1 cup | 380 | 2.0 | 1.0 | 0.0 | 50.0 | 8.0 |
| Triple cheese, from mix | 1 cup | 220 | 4.5 | 2.5 | 0.0 | 39.0 | 6.0 |
| Meatloaf, prepared w/beef, homemade | 6 oz. | 364 | 21.8 | 7.8 | n/a | 10.8 | n/a |
| Prepared w/turkey | 6 oz. | 290 | 10.3 | 3.0 | n/a | 12.5 | n/a |
| *■ Prepared w/ground turkey | 1 serv. | 175 | 3.0 | 0.6 | 0.0 | n/a | n/a |
| prepared w/beef substitute, vegetarian | 6 oz. | 335 | 15.3 | 2.4 | n/a | 13.6 | 2.0 |

■ Contains less than 20% fat
n/a Not available

* See note, page xli

| Item | SERVING | CAL-ORIES | FAT GRAMS | SAT. FAT GRAMS | TRANS FAT GRAMS | CARB. GRAMS | SUGAR GRAMS |
|---|---|---|---|---|---|---|---|
| Pepper steak, homemade | 3 oz. | 125 | 8.0 | 1.5 | n/a | 2.3 | 0.8 |
| ■ Ravioli, beef w/tomato & meat sauce, Chef Boyardee | 1 each | 229 | 5.4 | 2.5 | 0.0 | 36.9 | 5.3 |
| Spaghetti | | | | | | | |
| w/tomato sauce & cheese homemade | 1 cup | 260 | 8.8 | 2.0 | n/a | 37.0 | n/a |
| ■ Franco American | 1 cup | 210 | 2.0 | 1.0 | n/a | 40.0 | 14.0 |
| w/meat sauce, from mix, Spaghetti Classics | 1 cup | 330 | 10.0 | 3.5 | n/a | 47.0 | 7.0 |
| SpaghettiOs, Campbell's | 1 cup | 180 | 1.0 | 0.5 | n/a | 37.0 | 13 |
| w/meatballs | 1 cup | 240 | 8.0 | 3.5 | 0.5 | 32.0 | 11.0 |
| Taco, homemade | 1 small | 369 | 20.6 | 11.4 | n/a | 26.7 | n/a |
| * Tamale pie | 1 serv. | 352 | 4.8 | 0.9 | 0.0 | n/a | n/a |
| Tuna Helper, creamy noodle casserole | 1 cup | 300 | 14.0 | n/a | n/a | 30.0 | n/a |
| Veggie burger | | | | | | | |
| ■ Patty mix, Loma Linda | 1/3 cup | 91 | 1.0 | 0.2 | 0.0 | 6.6 | 0.4 |
| Redi Burger, Loma Linda, canned | 1 slice | 172 | 9.7 | 1.5 | 0.0 | 6.7 | 1.0 |
| Veggie weiner | | | | | | | |
| Big Franks, Loma Linda | 1 each | 118 | 7.1 | 0.8 | 0.0 | 1.5 | 0.2 |

## RICE & GRAINS

| Item | SERVING | CAL-ORIES | FAT GRAMS | SAT. FAT GRAMS | TRANS FAT GRAMS | CARB. GRAMS | SUGAR GRAMS |
|---|---|---|---|---|---|---|---|
| **Rice** | | | | | | | |
| ■ Arborio/risotto, dry | 2 oz. | 162 | 0.3 | 0.1 | 0.0 | 35.1 | 0.1 |
| ■ Brown, cooked | 1 cup | 218 | 1.6 | 0.3 | 0.0 | 45.8 | n/a |
| ■ Basmati, brown, dry, Arrowhead | 2 oz. | 189 | 2.0 | 0.0 | 0.0 | 41.9 | 1.4 |
| Quick, Spanish flavor, Lundberg Farms, dry | 1 serv. | 258 | 1.8 | 0.4 | 0.0 | 54.7 | 3.5 |
| ■ Dry Mix, Rice-A-Roni, chicken flavor, cooked | 1 cup | 310 | 1.0 | 0.0 | 0.0 | 51.0 | 2.0 |
| ■ 1/3 less salt | 2.5 oz. | 248 | 1.3 | 0.2 | 0.0 | 53.2 | 2.1 |
| ■ Near East, black beans/rice, Mediterranean | 2 oz. | 186 | 0.7 | 0.1 | 0.0 | 41.6 | 0.9 |
| ■ Curry | 2 oz. | 189 | 0.7 | 0.2 | 0.0 | 42.0 | 0.6 |
| ■ Spanish, homemade | 1 cup | 216 | 3.7 | 0.6 | 0.0 | 41.8 | n/a |
| ■ Lipton Fiesta Sides | 1/2 cup | 240 | 1.0 | 0.0 | 0.0 | 51.0 | 3.0 |
| ■ Rice-A-Roni, Spanish flavor | 1 cup | 300 | 1.0 | 0.0 | 0.0 | 41.0 | 3.0 |
| ■ White, cooked | 1 cup | 242 | 0.4 | 0.1 | 0.0 | 53.2 | 0.9 |
| Instant, Minute Rice | 1 cup | 160 | 0.0 | 0.0 | 0.0 | 36.0 | 0.0 |
| ■ Wild, cooked | 1 cup | 166 | 0.6 | 0.1 | 0.0 | 35.0 | 1.2 |
| Uncle Ben's, dry | 2 oz. | 200 | 1.3 | 0.0 | 0.0 | 42.5 | n/a |
| **Other Grains** | | | | | | | |
| ■ Barley, whole, cooked | 1 cup | 270 | 2.2 | 0.4 | 0.0 | 59.4 | n/a |
| ■ Pearled, cooked | 1 cup | 193 | 0.7 | 0.1 | 0.0 | 44.0 | n/a |

■ Contains less than 20% fat
n/a Not available

* See note, page xli

| Item | SERVING | CAL-ORIES | FAT GRAMS | SAT. FAT GRAMS | TRANS FAT GRAMS | CARB. GRAMS | SUGAR GRAMS |
|---|---|---|---|---|---|---|---|
| ■ Bulgur, cooked | 1 cup | 151 | 0.4 | 0.1 | 0.0 | 33.8 | 0.2 |
| ■ Couscous, cooked | 1 cup | 176 | 0.3 | 0.1 | 0.0 | 36.5 | 0.2 |
| ■ Near East, Parmesan Cheese flavor, dry | 2 oz. | 199 | 1.5 | 0.6 | 0.0 | 40.5 | 2.9 |
| ■ Kasha, roasted, cooked | 1 cup | 155 | 1.0 | 0.2 | 0.0 | 33.5 | 1.5 |
| ■ Millet, cooked | 1 cup | 207 | 1.7 | 0.3 | 0.0 | 41.2 | 0.2 |
| ■ Quinoa, dry | 2 oz. | 212 | 3.3 | 0.3 | 0.0 | 39.1 | n/a |
| ■ Spelt/caro, dry | 2 oz. | 211 | 1.6 | 0.0 | 0.0 | 40.5 | 0.0 |

## SALADS & SALAD BAR ITEMS

| Item | SERVING | CAL-ORIES | FAT GRAMS | SAT. FAT GRAMS | TRANS FAT GRAMS | CARB. GRAMS | SUGAR GRAMS |
|---|---|---|---|---|---|---|---|
| Almonds | 2 tb. | 103 | 9.0 | 0.7 | 0.0 | 3.5 | 0.9 |
| ■ Artichoke hearts | 3 pieces | 30 | 0.0 | 0.0 | 0.0 | 5.0 | 0.0 |
| Baba ghanoush | 2 oz. | 81 | 5.3 | n/a | 0.0 | 5.1 | n/a |
| Bacon bits, imitation | 2 tb. | 48 | 2.6 | 0.9 | 0.0 | 0.4 | 0.4 |
| ■ Beans, garbanzo, cooked | 2 tb. | 34 | 0.5 | 0.1 | 0.0 | 5.6 | 1.0 |
| ■ Bean sprouts, mung | 2 tb. | 4 | 0.0 | 0.0 | 0.0 | 0.8 | 0.5 |
| ■ Beets, shredded | 2 tb. | 8 | 0.0 | 0.0 | 0.0 | 1.8 | 1.3 |
| ■ Broccoli, florets | 2 tb. | 2 | 0.0 | 0.0 | 0.0 | 0.5 | 0.0 |
| ■ Cabbage, red, chopped | 1/2 cup | 14 | 0.1 | 0.0 | 0.0 | 3.3 | 1.7 |
| ■ Carrots, grated | 2 tb. | 6 | 0.0 | 0.0 | 0.0 | 1.3 | 0.6 |
| Carrot raisin, w/mayonnaise | 1/2 cup | 190 | 13.0 | 2.5 | n/a | 20.0 | 16.0 |
| Cheese, cheddar, shredded | 2 tb. | 57 | 4.7 | 3.0 | n/a | 0.2 | 0.1 |
| Cottage | 2 tb. | 25 | 1.1 | 0.8 | n/a | 1.0 | 1.0 |
| Chef salad, w/turkey, ham, & cheese, no dressing | 1.5 cups | 267 | 16.1 | 8.2 | n/a | 4.7 | n/a |
| ■ Chicken breast, diced, grilled | 2 oz. | 67 | 1.3 | n/a | n/a | 0.7 | n/a |
| Chicken, w/mayonnaise | 1/2 cup | 250 | 20.0 | 4.0 | n/a | 9.0 | 4.0 |
| Coleslaw | 6 oz. | 150 | 8.0 | n/a | 0.0 | 18.0 | n/a |
| Croutons | 2 tb. | 23 | 0.9 | 0.3 | n/a | 3.2 | 0.8 |
| ■ Cucumbers | 2 pieces | 2 | 0.0 | 0.0 | 0.0 | 0.3 | 0.2 |
| Earthbound Farm, Organic | | | | | | | |
| Arugula Salad | 2 cups | 15 | 0.5 | 0.0 | 0.0 | 3.0 | 0.0 |
| ■ Baby Romaine | 2 cups | 15 | 0.0 | 0.0 | 0.0 | 3.0 | 0.0 |
| ■ Fresh Herb | 2 cups | 15 | 0.0 | 0.0 | 0.0 | 4.0 | 0.0 |
| ■ Mixed Baby Greens | 2 cups | 15 | 0.0 | 0.0 | 0.0 | 4.0 | 0.0 |
| Grab & Go w/vinaigrette & walnuts | 1.5 cups | 220 | 23.0 | 3.0 | 0.0 | 3.0 | 0.0 |
| ■ Savory Spinach | 2 cups | 10 | 0.0 | 0.0 | 0.0 | 6.0 | 0.0 |
| Eggs, hard boiled, chopped | 2 tb. | 27 | 1.8 | 0.6 | 0.0 | 0.2 | 0.2 |
| ■ Fruit salad | 1/2 cup | 45 | 0.0 | 0.0 | 0.0 | 10.6 | 9.3 |
| ■ Hummus | 2 tb. | 52 | 3.0 | 0.5 | 0.0 | 4.5 | n/a |
| ■ Lettuce | 1 cup | 7 | 0.1 | 0.0 | 0.0 | 1.2 | 0.5 |
| Lobster w/mayonnaise | 1/2 cup | 75 | 3.8 | 0.7 | n/a | 5.1 | n/a |
| ■ Mushrooms, raw | 1/4 cup | 4 | 0.1 | 0.0 | 0.0 | 0.6 | 0.3 |
| ■ Onion, red, chopped | 2 tb. | 8 | 0.0 | 0.0 | 0.0 | 2.0 | 0.9 |
| ■ Palm hearts | 2 tb. | 5 | 0.1 | 0.0 | 0.0 | 0.8 | n/a |
| Pasta w/Italian dressing | 1/2 cup | 136 | 6.1 | 0.8 | n/a | 17.4 | 2.3 |

■ Contains less than 20% fat
n/a Not available

| Item | SERVING | CAL-ORIES | FAT GRAMS | SAT. FAT GRAMS | TRANS FAT GRAMS | CARB. GRAMS | SUGAR GRAMS |
|---|---|---|---|---|---|---|---|
| * ■ Pasta w/seafood | 1 cup | 243 | 1.8 | 0.3 | 0.0 | n/a | n/a |
| ■ Peppers, bell, green, sweet, strips | 2 pieces | 1 | 0.0 | 0.0 | 0.0 | 0.3 | 0.1 |
| ■ Roasted | 1/2 cup | 30 | 0.0 | 0.0 | 0.0 | 5.0 | 4.0 |
| Potato, w/mayonnaise and hard-boiled egg | 1/2 cup | 152 | 8.3 | 1.1 | n/a | 18.9 | 6.8 |
| ■ Potato, German | 1/2 cup | 120 | 3.0 | 0.2 | 0.0 | 22.0 | 8.5 |
| Pumpkin seeds | 2 tb. | 93 | 7.9 | 1.5 | 0.0 | 3.1 | 0.2 |
| ■ Radishes, slices | 2 tb. | 2 | 0.0 | 0.0 | 0.0 | 0.3 | n/a |
| Sunflower seeds | 2 tb. | 120 | 10.0 | 1.0 | 0.0 | 3.3 | 0.7 |
| Tabbouleh | 1/2 cup | 100 | 7.5 | 1.0 | 0.0 | 8.0 | n/a |
| Tofu | 1/2 cup | 94 | 5.9 | 0.9 | 0.0 | 2.3 | 0.5 |
| Three bean, w/oil dressing | 1/2 cup | 70 | 3.8 | 0.6 | 0.0 | 7.5 | n/a |
| ■ Tomatoes, red, fresh, chopped | 2 tb. | 5 | 0.1 | 0.0 | 0.0 | 1.0 | 0.6 |
| Tuna w/mayonnaise | 1/2 cup | 260 | 19.0 | 3.0 | n/a | 9.0 | 4.0 |
| ■ Tuna, light, packed in water | 2 oz. | 70 | 0.1 | 0.0 | 0.0 | 0.0 | 0.0 |
| Turkey w/mayonnaise | 1/2 cup | 170 | 11.0 | 3.0 | n/a | 12.0 | 6.0 |
| Waldorf, prepared from recipe | 1/2 cup | 206 | 20.4 | 2.1 | n/a | 5.9 | 3.1 |
| Walnuts, chopped | 2 tb. | 98 | 9.8 | 0.9 | 0.0 | 2.1 | 0.4 |

## SALAD DRESSINGS

| Item | SERVING | CAL-ORIES | FAT GRAMS | SAT. FAT GRAMS | TRANS FAT GRAMS | CARB. GRAMS | SUGAR GRAMS |
|---|---|---|---|---|---|---|---|
| Blue cheese | | | | | | | |
| Girard's, Vinaigrette | 2 tb. | 100 | 10.0 | 2.0 | 0.0 | 3.0 | 3.0 |
| ■ Kraft Free | 2 tb. | 45 | 0.0 | 0.0 | 0.0 | 11.0 | 2.0 |
| Nancy's Healthy Kitchen Light | 2 tb. | 30 | 1.5 | 1.0 | 0.0 | 2.0 | 1.0 |
| Caesar | | | | | | | |
| ■ Kraft Free | 2 tb. | 45 | 0.0 | 0.0 | 0.0 | 11.0 | 2.0 |
| Marie's | 2 tb. | 250 | 25.0 | 4.0 | n/a | 6.0 | 0.5 |
| Seven Seas | 2 tb. | 100 | 10.0 | 1.5 | n/a | 2.0 | 1.0 |
| Walden Farms | 2 tb. | 0 | 0.0 | 0.0 | 0.0 | 0.0 | 0.0 |
| Champagne, Light, Girard's | 2 tb. | 60 | 5.0 | 1.0 | 0.0 | 2.0 | 1.0 |
| Chinese Chicken, Joey D's | 2 tb. | 120 | 11.0 | 1.5 | 0.0 | 5.0 | 5.0 |
| Coleslaw, Marie's | 2 tb. | 150 | 13.0 | 2.0 | n/a | 6.0 | 6.0 |
| French | | | | | | | |
| Good Seasons, honey, from mix | 2 tb. | 160 | 15.0 | 2.0 | 0.0 | 5.0 | 4.0 |
| ■ Fat free | 2 tb. | 20 | 0.0 | 0.0 | 0.0 | 5.0 | 4.0 |
| Kraft | 2 tb. | 160 | 15.0 | 2.6 | 0.0 | 5.0 | 5.0 |
| ■ Kraft Free | 2 tb. | 45 | 0.0 | 0.0 | 0.0 | 11.0 | 5.0 |
| Marie's | 2 tb. | 130 | 11.0 | 1.5 | n/a | 8.0 | 7.0 |
| Wishbone | 2 tb. | 130 | 12.0 | 2.0 | 0.0 | 6.0 | 5.0 |
| Just 2 Good! | 2 tb. | 50 | 2.0 | 0.0 | 0.0 | 9.0 | 5.0 |
| Green Goddess | 2 tb. | 130 | 13.0 | 2.0 | n/a | 1.0 | 1.0 |
| Italian, creamy | | | | | | | |
| Kraft | 2 tb. | 110 | 11.0 | 1.5 | 0.0 | 2.0 | 2.0 |
| ■ Kraft Free | 2 tb. | 50 | 0.0 | 0.0 | 0.0 | 12.0 | 4.0 |
| Seven Seas | 2 tb. | 120 | 12.0 | 2.0 | 0.0 | 1.0 | 1.0 |
| 1/3 less fat | 2 tb. | 60 | 5.0 | 1.0 | 0.0 | 2.0 | 2.0 |

■ Contains less than 20% fat
n/a Not available

* See note, page xli

| Item | SERVING | CAL-ORIES | FAT GRAMS | SAT. FAT GRAMS | TRANS FAT GRAMS | CARB. GRAMS | SUGAR GRAMS |
|---|---|---|---|---|---|---|---|
| ■ Fat free | 2 tb. | 50 | 0.0 | 0.0 | 0.0 | 12.0 | 4.0 |
| Italian, regular | | | | | | | |
| Bernstein's Italian | 2 tb. | 130 | 11.0 | 0.5 | 0.0 | 8.0 | 5.0 |
| Good Seasons, reduced calorie, from mix | 2 tb. | 50 | 5.0 | 1.0 | 0.0 | 2.0 | 1.0 |
| ■ Fat free | 2 tb. | 10 | 0.0 | 0.0 | 0.0 | 3.0 | 2.0 |
| Zesty | 2 tb. | 70 | 7.5 | 1.0 | 0.0 | 0.5 | 0.5 |
| Reduced calorie | 2 tb. | 50 | 5.0 | 1.0 | 0.0 | 3.0 | 2.0 |
| Kraft, Zesty | 2 tb. | 109 | 11.1 | 1.2 | 0.0 | 1.8 | 1.3 |
| Kraft, ⅓ less fat | 2 tb. | 70 | 7.0 | 1.0 | 0.0 | 3.0 | 2.0 |
| ■ Kraft Free | 2 tb. | 20 | 0.3 | 0.2 | 0.0 | 3.6 | 2.2 |
| ■ Marie's Italian vinaigrette, fat free | 2 tb. | 35 | 0.0 | 0.0 | 0.0 | 8.0 | 4.0 |
| Newman's Own Lemon Light Italian | 2 tb. | 60 | 6.0 | 1.0 | 0.0 | 0.0 | 0.0 |
| Seven Seas, w/olive oil blend, reduced fat | 2 tb. | 45 | 4.0 | 0.0 | 0.0 | 2.0 | 2.0 |
| Tomato & herb | 2 tb. | 100 | 9.0 | 1.0 | 0.0 | 3.0 | 3.0 |
| Viva | 2 tb. | 90 | 9.0 | 1.0 | 0.0 | 2.0 | 1.0 |
| ⅓ less fat, Viva | 2 tb. | 45 | 4.0 | 0.0 | 0.0 | 2.0 | 1.0 |
| ■ Walden Farms Sugar Free Italian Dressing w/Soy Protein | 2 tb. | 15 | 0.0 | 0.0 | 0.0 | 1.0 | 0.0 |
| ■ Mango, Consorzio, Fat Free | 2 tb. | 30 | 0.0 | 0.0 | 0.0 | 8.0 | 6.0 |
| Mayonnaise, Best Food/Hellman's | 1 tb. | 100 | 11.0 | 1.5 | 0.0 | 0.0 | 0.0 |
| Reduced fat, Just 2 Good! | 1 tb. | 25 | 2.0 | 0.0 | 0.0 | 2.0 | 1.0 |
| Light, Smart Balance | 1 tb. | 50 | 5.0 | 0.0 | 0.0 | 2.0 | n/a |
| Light, Kraft | 1 tb. | 50 | 4.9 | 0.8 | 0.0 | 1.3 | 0.6 |
| Fat free | 1 tb. | 11 | 0.4 | 0.1 | 0.0 | 2.0 | 1.1 |
| Mayonnaise substitute, Nayonaise | 1 tb. | 35 | 3.5 | 0.5 | 0.0 | 1.0 | 0.0 |
| Miracle Whip | 1 tb. | 70 | 7.0 | 1.0 | 0.0 | 2.0 | 1.0 |
| Light | 1 tb. | 37 | 3.0 | 0.5 | 0.0 | 2.3 | 1.6 |
| Fat free | 1 tb. | 13 | 0.4 | 0.1 | 0.0 | 2.5 | 1.7 |
| Ranch | | | | | | | |
| Hidden Valley | 2 tb. | 140 | 14.0 | 1.5 | 0.0 | 1.0 | 1.0 |
| Hidden Valley, light | 2 tb. | 80 | 7.0 | 1.0 | 0.0 | 3.0 | 1.0 |
| Kraft | 2 tb. | 148 | 15.6 | 2.4 | 0.0 | 1.3 | 1.2 |
| ■ Kraft Free | 2 tb. | 48 | 0.4 | 0.1 | 0.0 | 10.7 | 2.1 |
| Marie's, zesty, low fat | 2 tb. | 45 | 1.5 | 0.0 | n/a | 7.0 | 3.0 |
| Creamy, reduced calorie | 2 tb. | 100 | 7.0 | 0.5 | n/a | 7.0 | 3.0 |
| Seven Seas | 2 tb. | 160 | 17.0 | 2.5 | n/a | 2.0 | 1.0 |
| ⅓ less fat | 2 tb. | 100 | 9.0 | 1.5 | n/a | 5.0 | 2.0 |
| ■ Fat free | 2 tb. | 45 | 0.0 | 0.0 | 0.0 | 11.0 | 2.0 |
| T. Marzetti, Parmesan Ranch | 2 tb. | 140 | 14.0 | 2.0 | 0.0 | 2.0 | 1.0 |
| Russian | 2 tb. | 130 | 10.0 | 1.5 | n/a | 10.0 | 10.0 |
| Sesame Seed | 2 tb. | 136 | 13.8 | 2.0 | n/a | 2.6 | 2.4 |
| Thousand Island, Kraft | 2 tb. | 110 | 10.0 | 1.5 | n/a | 5.0 | 4.0 |

■ Contains less than 20% fat
n/a Not available

| Item | SERVING | CAL-ORIES | FAT GRAMS | SAT. FAT GRAMS | TRANS FAT GRAMS | CARB. GRAMS | SUGAR GRAMS |
|---|---|---|---|---|---|---|---|
| ⅓ less fat | 2 tb. | 70 | 4.5 | 0.5 | n/a | 7.0 | 5.0 |
| ■ Kraft Free | 2 tb. | 40 | 0.0 | 0.0 | 0.0 | 9.0 | 5.0 |
| Vinaigrette | | | | | | | |
| Girard's Balsamic Basil | 2 tb. | 90 | 9.0 | 1.5 | 0.0 | 3.0 | 2.0 |
| ■ Marie's, classic herb, fat free | 2 tb. | 30 | 0.0 | 0.0 | 0.0 | 7.0 | 3.0 |
| ■ Marukan Seasoned Gourmet Rice Vinegar | 2 tb. | 50 | 0.0 | 0.0 | 0.0 | 12.5 | n/a |
| Newman's Own Light Balsamic Vinaigrette | 2 tb. | 45 | 4.0 | 0.5 | 0.0 | 2.0 | 1.0 |
| Seven Seas, herb | 2 tb. | 140 | 15.0 | 2.0 | n/a | 1.0 | 0.0 |
| ■ Raspberry, fat free | 2 tb. | 30 | 0.0 | 0.0 | 0.0 | 7.0 | 7.0 |

## SAUCES & GRAVIES

| Item | SERVING | CAL-ORIES | FAT GRAMS | SAT. FAT GRAMS | TRANS FAT GRAMS | CARB. GRAMS | SUGAR GRAMS |
|---|---|---|---|---|---|---|---|
| A.1. Steak Sauce | 1 tb. | 15 | 0.0 | 0.0 | 0.0 | 3.0 | 2.0 |
| Alfredo, Buitoni, refrigerated | ¼ cup | 140 | 12.0 | 7.0 | 0.0 | 5.0 | 2.0 |
| Alfredo, Light, Buitoni, refrigerated | ¼ cup | 95 | 6.5 | 3.5 | 0.0 | 5.0 | 2.5 |
| ■ BBQ, Open Pit, original flavor | 2 tb. | 50 | 0.0 | 0.0 | 0.0 | 11.0 | 9.0 |
| ■ Chili sauce | 2 tb. | 40 | 0.0 | 0.0 | 0.0 | 10.0 | 8.0 |
| Chinese marinade, Soy Vay | 1 tb. | 40 | 1.0 | 0.0 | 0.0 | 7.0 | 7.0 |
| ■ Chutney, homemade | 2 tb. | 52 | 0.2 | 0.0 | 0.0 | 13.4 | 11.9 |
| ■ Wax Orchards, apricot ginger, low sodium | 2 tb. | 50 | 0.5 | n/a | 0.0 | 11.0 | 10.0 |
| ■ Cranberry, low sodium | 2 tb. | 50 | 0.5 | n/a | 0.0 | 11.0 | 10.0 |
| ■ Patak's Major Grey's Mango Chutney | 1 tb. | 50 | 0.0 | 0.0 | 0.0 | 12.0 | 12.0 |
| Clam, white, Progresso | ½ cup | 150 | 10.0 | 1.5 | 0.0 | 5.0 | 1.0 |
| ■ Red, Progresso | ½ cup | 60 | 1.0 | 0.0 | 0.0 | 8.0 | 4.0 |
| ■ Cranberry sauce, canned | ½ cup | 209 | 0.2 | 0.0 | 0.0 | 53.9 | 52.5 |
| ■ Jellied | ½ cup | 200 | 0.0 | 0.0 | 0.0 | 52.0 | 34.0 |
| ■ Fish sauce | 1 tb. | 6 | 0.0 | 0.0 | 0.0 | 0.7 | 0.0 |
| ■ Hoisin sauce | 1 tb. | 30 | 0.0 | 0.0 | 0.0 | 9.0 | 6.0 |
| Hollandaise, homemade | 2 tb. | 85 | 9.1 | 5.1 | n/a | 0.3 | n/a |
| ■ Knorr, from dry mix | 2 tb. | 10 | 0.0 | 0.0 | 0.0 | 2.0 | 0.0 |
| ■ Oyster sauce | 1 tb. | 2 | 0.0 | 0.0 | 0.0 | 0.4 | 0.0 |
| Pesto | 2 tb. | 155 | 14.2 | 3.8 | 0.0 | 2.0 | n/a |
| ■ Picante, medium, Ortega | 2 tb. | 10 | 0.0 | 0.0 | 0.0 | 2.0 | 0.0 |
| ■ Plum sauce | 1 tb. | 35 | 0.2 | 0.0 | 0.0 | 8.2 | n/a |
| Pizza Sauce, Ragu | 2 tb. | 15 | 0.5 | 0.0 | 0.0 | 2.0 | 1.5 |
| ■ Relish, cranberry orange | ½ cup | 245 | 0.1 | 0.0 | 0.0 | 63.5 | n/a |
| ■ Salsa | 2 tb. | 10 | 0.0 | 0.0 | 0.0 | 2.0 | 1.0 |
| ■ Guiltless Gourmet, Southwestern Grill | 2 tb. | 10 | 0.0 | 0.0 | 0.0 | 2.0 | 1.0 |
| Pasta sauce w/meat | | | | | | | |
| Prego, meat | ½ cup | 130 | 5.0 | 1.0 | 0.0 | 19.0 | 12.0 |
| Progresso, meat | ½ cup | 100 | 4.5 | 1.0 | 0.0 | 12.0 | 9.0 |
| Ragu, meat, Classic Italian | ½ cup | 150 | 10.0 | 3.0 | 0.0 | 9.0 | 6.0 |

■ Contains less than 20% fat
n/a Not available

| Item | SERVING | CAL-ORIES | FAT GRAMS | SAT. FAT GRAMS | TRANS FAT GRAMS | CARB. GRAMS | SUGAR GRAMS |
|---|---|---|---|---|---|---|---|
| Pasta sauce, meatless | | | | | | | |
| Campbell's | 1/2 cup | 110 | 3.0 | 0.5 | 0.0 | 19.0 | 13.0 |
| ■ DiGiorno, plum tomato & mushroom | 1/2 cup | 60 | 0.0 | 0.0 | 0.0 | 13.0 | 10.0 |
| ■ Muir Glen, organic, chunky | 1/2 cup | 40 | 0.0 | 0.0 | 0.0 | 8.0 | 4.0 |
| ■ Balsamic Roasted Onion | 1/2 cup | 50 | 0.5 | 0.0 | 0.0 | 12.0 | 5.0 |
| Four Cheese | 1/2 cup | 80 | 2.5 | 1.0 | 0.0 | 11.0 | 3.0 |
| ■ Italian Herb | 1/2 cup | 55 | 0.5 | 0.0 | 0.0 | 12.0 | 5.0 |
| ■ No salt added | 1/2 cup | 40 | 0.0 | 0.0 | 0.0 | 10.0 | 6.0 |
| Newman's Own Sockarooni | 1/2 cup | 60 | 2.0 | 0.0 | 0.0 | 9.0 | 7.0 |
| ■ Ragu, tomato & basil, light | 1/2 cup | 50 | 0.0 | 0.0 | 0.0 | 10.0 | 8.0 |
| Ragu, marinara, Old World Style | 1/2 cup | 80 | 4.5 | 0.5 | 0.0 | 11.0 | 7.0 |
| Trader Joe's, marinara, Tomato Basil, Low fat | 1/2 cup | 60 | 3.0 | 0.0 | 0.0 | 8.0 | 3.0 |
| ■ Soy, Kikkoman | 1 tb. | 10 | 0.0 | 0.0 | 0.0 | 0.0 | 0.0 |
| ■ Light | 1 tb. | 10 | 0.0 | 0.0 | 0.0 | 1.0 | 0.0 |
| ■ Stir Fry Sauce, General Tsao, Trader Joe's | 1/4 cup | 130 | 0.0 | 0.0 | 0.0 | 33.0 | 29.0 |
| ■ Stroganoff, beef, from dry mix | 3 oz. | 240 | 0.0 | 0.0 | 0.0 | 48.0 | n/a |
| Tabasco | 1 tb. | 2 | 0.1 | 0.0 | 0.0 | 0.1 | n/a |
| ■ Tamari, regular & reduced sodium | 1 tb. | 15 | 0.0 | 0.0 | 0.0 | 1.0 | n/a |
| Tartar, Kraft | 2 tb. | 90 | 9.0 | 1.5 | n/a | 4.0 | 2.0 |
| ■ Teriyaki | 2 tb. | 30 | 0.0 | 0.0 | 0.0 | 5.7 | 3.5 |
| Veri Veri | 2 tb. | 35 | 1.0 | 0.0 | 0.0 | 6.0 | 5.0 |
| Thai Peanut Sauce, Trader Joe's | 2 tb. | 50 | 3.0 | 1.0 | 0.0 | 5.0 | 3.0 |
| White, Knorr, from dry mix | 2 tb. | 13 | 0.5 | 0.3 | 0.0 | 2.0 | 0.5 |
| ■ Worcestershire | 1 tb. | 15 | 0.0 | n/a | 0.0 | 3.4 | 2.5 |
| ■ Low sodium, Angostura | 1 tb. | 5 | 0.0 | 0.0 | 0.0 | 1.0 | 1.0 |
| | | | | | | | |
| **Gravies** | | | | | | | |
| ■ Au jus, Franco-American | 1/4 cup | 5 | 0.0 | 0.0 | 0.0 | 0.0 | 0.0 |
| Beef, Franco-American | 2 tb. | 13 | 0.5 | 0.3 | 0.0 | 1.5 | 0.5 |
| Brown, Heinz | 2 tb. | 12 | 0.4 | 0.2 | 0.0 | 1.7 | n/a |
| Brown, Knorr, Classic, from dry mix | 1/4 tb. | 1 | 0.0 | 0.0 | 0.0 | 0.2 | 0.1 |
| Chicken, canned | 2 tb. | 18 | 1.0 | 0.5 | 0.0 | 2.0 | 0.5 |
| ■ Fat free | 2 tb. | 8 | 0.0 | 0.0 | 0.0 | 1.5 | 0.5 |
| ■ Chicken, Knorr, from dry mix | 2 tb. | 13 | 0.3 | 0.0 | 0.0 | 2.0 | 0.5 |
| Mushroom, Franco-American | 2 tb. | 10 | 0.5 | 0.0 | 0.0 | 1.5 | 0.5 |
| Knorr | 2 tb. | 10 | 0.3 | 0.0 | 0.0 | 1.5 | 0.5 |
| ■ Pork, Knorr, from dry mix | 2 tb. | 13 | 0.0 | 0.0 | 0.0 | 2.0 | 0.5 |
| Turkey, Franco-American | 2 tb. | 10 | 0.3 | 0.0 | 0.0 | 2.0 | 0.0 |
| ■ Fat free | 2 tb. | 10 | 0.0 | 0.0 | 0.0 | 2.0 | 0.0 |
| ■ Turkey, from dry mix | 2 tb. | 13 | 0.3 | 0.0 | 0.0 | 2.0 | 0.5 |

■ Contains less than 20% fat
n/a Not available

| Item | SERVING | CAL-ORIES | FAT GRAMS | SAT. FAT GRAMS | TRANS FAT GRAMS | CARB. GRAMS | SUGAR GRAMS |
|---|---|---|---|---|---|---|---|

## SNACKS

**Corn Chips**

| Item | SERVING | CAL-ORIES | FAT GRAMS | SAT. FAT GRAMS | TRANS FAT GRAMS | CARB. GRAMS | SUGAR GRAMS |
|---|---|---|---|---|---|---|---|
| Fritos | 1 oz. | 160 | 10.0 | 1.0 | 0.0 | 15.0 | 0.0 |
| Tortilla chips | | | | | | | |
|    Doritos, Nacho Cheesier | 1 oz. | 140 | 7.0 | 1.5 | 0.0 | 17.0 | 2.0 |
| ■  Guiltless Gourmet, yellow corn | 1 oz. | 111 | 2.0 | 0.0 | 0.0 | 22.3 | 0.0 |
| ■    Blue corn | 1 oz. | 111 | 2.0 | 0.0 | 0.0 | 22.3 | 0.0 |
| ■    Unsalted | 1 oz. | 111 | 1.0 | 0.0 | 0.0 | 22.3 | 0.0 |
|    Tostitos, Hint of Lime | 1 oz. | 140 | 6.0 | 1.0 | 0.0 | 18.0 | 1.0 |

**Dips**

| Item | SERVING | CAL-ORIES | FAT GRAMS | SAT. FAT GRAMS | TRANS FAT GRAMS | CARB. GRAMS | SUGAR GRAMS |
|---|---|---|---|---|---|---|---|
| Artichoke Lemon Pesto, Bella Cucina | 1/4 cup | 140 | 12.0 | 1.5 | 0.0 | 5.0 | 0.0 |
| Avocado, Kraft | 2 tb. | 60 | 4.0 | 3.0 | 0.0 | 4.0 | 1.0 |
| Bacon & horseradish, Kraft | 2 tb. | 60 | 5.0 | 3.0 | n/a | 3.0 | 1.0 |
| Bean, Fritos | 2 tb. | 40 | 1.0 | 0.0 | 0.0 | 5.0 | 0.0 |
| ■ Bean, black, mild, Guiltless Gourmet | 2 tb. | 30 | 0.0 | 0.0 | 0.0 | 5.0 | 1.0 |
| Sour cream, bacon, & onion, Kraft | 2 tb. | 60 | 5.0 | 3.0 | 0.0 | 2.0 | 1.0 |
| Clam, Kraft | 2 tb. | 60 | 4.0 | 3.0 | 0.0 | 3.0 | 1.0 |
| Guacamole | 2 tb. | 29 | 2.0 | 0.0 | 0.0 | 2.0 | n/a |
| Nacho Beef, Fiesta, Ortega, frozen | 2 tb. | 60 | 3.5 | 1.5 | 0.0 | 4.0 | 1.0 |
| Onion, French, Kraft | 2 tb. | 60 | 4.0 | 3.0 | n/a | 4.0 | 1.0 |
| ■  Fat free | 2 tb. | 25 | 0.0 | 0.0 | 0.0 | 4.0 | 2.0 |
| Ranch, T. Marzetti | 2 tb. | 120 | 12.0 | 3.5 | 0.0 | 2.0 | 1.0 |
| ■  Fat free | 2 tb. | 25 | 0.0 | 0.0 | 0.0 | 4.0 | 2.0 |
| Salsa con Queso, Tostitos | 2 tb. | 40 | 2.5 | 1.0 | 0.0 | 5.0 | 0.5 |
| ■ Salsa, Garden Pepper, medium, Old El Paso | 2 tb. | 10 | 0.0 | 0.0 | 0.0 | 2.0 | 1.0 |
| Spinach, T. Marzetti | 2 tb. | 130 | 13.0 | 3.0 | 0.0 | 2.0 | 1.0 |

**Granola & Energy Bars**

| Item | SERVING | CAL-ORIES | FAT GRAMS | SAT. FAT GRAMS | TRANS FAT GRAMS | CARB. GRAMS | SUGAR GRAMS |
|---|---|---|---|---|---|---|---|
| Granola | | | | | | | |
|    Chocolate chip, chewy, Quaker Oats | 1 each | 77 | 2.5 | 1.0 | 0.0 | 13.2 | 6.0 |
|    Health Valley, Peanut Crunch, low fat, chewy | 1 each | 110 | 3.0 | 0.0 | 0.0 | 19.0 | 10.0 |
|    Oatmeal Raisin, cherry, Quaker Oats | 1 each | 90 | 1.5 | 0.0 | 0.0 | 19.0 | 7.0 |
|    Oats 'n Honey, Nature Valley | 1 each | 90 | 3.0 | 0.3 | 0.0 | 14.5 | 5.5 |
| ■  Strawberry Yogurt, Nature Valley | 1 each | 140 | 3.5 | 2.0 | 0.0 | 26.0 | 13.0 |

■ Contains less than 20% fat
n/a Not available

| Item | SERVING | CAL-ORIES | FAT GRAMS | SAT. FAT GRAMS | TRANS FAT GRAMS | CARB. GRAMS | SUGAR GRAMS |
|---|---|---|---|---|---|---|---|
| Trail mix, Fruit & Nut, chewy Energy | 1 each | 140 | 4.0 | 0.5 | 0.0 | 25.0 | 13.0 |
| Balance, Caramel Nut Blast | 1 each | 200 | 7.0 | 4.0 | 0.0 | 23.0 | 17.0 |
| ■ Clif, Black Cherry Almond | 1 each | 250 | 45.0 | 15.0 | 0.0 | 44.0 | 20.0 |
| Luna, Nutz Over Chocolate | 1 each | 173 | 4.4 | 2.7 | 0.0 | 25.3 | 12.1 |
| ■ Power, Apple Cinnamon | 1 each | 230 | 2.5 | 0.5 | 0.0 | 45.0 | 20.0 |

### Popcorn

| Item | SERVING | CAL-ORIES | FAT GRAMS | SAT. FAT GRAMS | TRANS FAT GRAMS | CARB. GRAMS | SUGAR GRAMS |
|---|---|---|---|---|---|---|---|
| ■ Air popped, no salt | 1 cup | 31 | 0.3 | 0.1 | 0.0 | 6.2 | 0.1 |
| Bagged, plain, Whole Foods | 3.5 cups | 140 | 5.0 | 0.0 | 0.0 | 21.0 | 0.0 |
| Buttered, Orville Redenbacher's Smart Pop | 1 cup | 15.0 | 2.0 | 0.5 | 0.0 | 26.0 | n/a |
| Buttered, Pop Secret | 1 cup | 35 | 12.0 | 3.0 | 0.0 | 17.0 | 0.0 |
| Light, Orville Redenbacher's | 1 cup | 22 | 1.0 | 0.2 | 0.0 | 3.8 | 0.0 |
| Oil popped | 1 cup | 55 | 3.1 | 0.5 | 0.0 | 6.3 | 0.1 |

### Potato Chips

| Item | SERVING | CAL-ORIES | FAT GRAMS | SAT. FAT GRAMS | TRANS FAT GRAMS | CARB. GRAMS | SUGAR GRAMS |
|---|---|---|---|---|---|---|---|
| Cape Cod | 1 oz. | 150 | 8.0 | 2.5 | 0.0 | 17.0 | 1.0 |
| 40% less fat | 1 oz. | 130 | 6.0 | 0.5 | 0.0 | 18.0 | 1.0 |
| Dirty, light salt | 1 oz. | 150 | 8.0 | 1.5 | 0.0 | 17.0 | 0.0 |
| ■ Kettle Krisps, low fat, lightly salted | 1 oz. | 110 | 1.5 | 0.0 | 0.0 | 22.0 | 0.0 |
| Lay's, Classic | 1 oz. | 150 | 10.0 | 3.0 | 0.0 | 15.0 | 0.0 |
| ■ Baked | 1 oz. | 110 | 1.5 | 0.0 | 0.0 | 23.0 | 2.0 |
| Salt & Vinegar | 1 oz. | 150 | 10.0 | 2.5 | 0.0 | 15.0 | 1.0 |
| Ruffles, Original | 1 oz. | 160 | 10.0 | 2.5 | 0.0 | 14.0 | 0.0 |
| Baked | 1 oz. | 130 | 3.0 | 0.0 | 0.0 | 24.0 | 2.0 |
| Reduced fat | 1 oz. | 130 | 6.7 | 1.0 | 0.0 | 18.0 | 0.0 |
| Pringle | 1 oz. | 160 | 11.0 | 3.0 | 0.0 | 15.0 | 0.0 |
| Reduced fat | 16 | 140 | 7.0 | 2.0 | 0.0 | 19.0 | 0.0 |
| Terra, Olive Oil & Fine Herb | 1 oz. | 140 | 7.0 | 1.0 | 0.0 | 18.0 | 1.0 |

### Pretzels

| Item | SERVING | CAL-ORIES | FAT GRAMS | SAT. FAT GRAMS | TRANS FAT GRAMS | CARB. GRAMS | SUGAR GRAMS |
|---|---|---|---|---|---|---|---|
| ■ Olde Tyme, Snyder's | 1 oz. | 120 | 1.0 | 0.0 | 0.0 | 24.0 | n/a |
| ■ Snaps, Snyders, 100 | ½ oz. | 100 | 0.5 | 0.0 | 0.0 | 22.0 | <1.0 |
| ■ Sourdough, Hard, Fat-free, Snyder's | 1 oz. | 100 | 0.0 | 0.0 | 0.0 | 22.0 | n/a |
| ■ Spelt, Newman's Own | 20 pieces | 120 | 1.0 | 0.0 | 0.0 | 23.0 | 0.0 |
| ■ Sticks, Laura Scudder, fat-free | 1 oz. | 110 | 0.0 | 0.0 | 0.0 | 25.0 | 1.0 |
| ■ Thin pretzels, Rold Gold | 9 pieces | 110 | 1.0 | 0.0 | 0.0 | 25.0 | 1.0 |
| ■ Tiny twists, Rold Gold, fat free | 1 oz. | 100 | 0.0 | 0.0 | 0.0 | 23.0 | 1.0 |
| ■ Unsalted, Hard, Snyder's | 1 oz. | 100 | 0.0 | 0.0 | 0.0 | 22.0 | n/a |

### Other Snacks

| Item | SERVING | CAL-ORIES | FAT GRAMS | SAT. FAT GRAMS | TRANS FAT GRAMS | CARB. GRAMS | SUGAR GRAMS |
|---|---|---|---|---|---|---|---|
| Bagel Chips | 1 oz. | 121 | 3.0 | 0.5 | 0.0 | 21.2 | n/a |
| Bugles | 1.3 cup | 160 | 9.0 | 8.0 | 0.0 | 18.0 | 1.0 |
| Chaos Chips | 1 oz. | 140 | 6.0 | 1.0 | 0.0 | 18.0 | 1.0 |

■ Contains less than 20% fat
n/a Not available

| Item | SERVING | CAL-ORIES | FAT GRAMS | SAT. FAT GRAMS | TRANS FAT GRAMS | CARB. GRAMS | SUGAR GRAMS |
|---|---|---|---|---|---|---|---|
| Cheese Puffs, Barbara's | 1 oz. | 150 | 10.0 | 1.5 | 0.0 | 16.0 | 0.0 |
| Cheetos | 1 oz. | 160 | 10.0 | 2.5 | 0.0 | 15.0 | 1.0 |
| Crunchy | 1 oz. | 160 | 10.0 | 2.5 | 0.0 | 15.0 | 1.0 |
| Corn Nuts | 1 oz. | 126 | 4.4 | 0.7 | 0.0 | 20.4 | 0.2 |
| ■ Cracker Jacks, Original | 1 oz. | 122 | 2.0 | 0.0 | 0.0 | 23.3 | 15.2 |
| ■ Caramel, fat free | 1 oz. | 111 | 0.0 | 0.0 | 0.0 | 26.3 | 17.2 |
| ■ Fruit Roll-Ups, Crazy Colors | 2 each | 104 | 1.1 | 0.5 | 0.0 | 23.8 | 10.4 |
| Pirate's Booty | 1 oz. | 130 | 5.0 | 1.0 | 0.0 | 18.0 | 0.0 |
| Pita Chips, Trader Joe's | 1 oz. | 130 | 4.0 | 0.0 | 0.0 | 18.0 | 2.0 |
| Pita Chips, Stacy's | 1 oz. | 130 | 4.0 | 0.0 | 0.0 | 18.0 | 2.0 |
| Pork Skins, plain | 1 oz. | 155 | 8.9 | 3.2 | 0.0 | 0.0 | 0.0 |
| Potato Sticks | 1 oz. | 149 | 9.0 | 1.5 | n/a | 15.3 | 0.2 |
| ■ Rice Cake, Quaker, Mini, Caramel Corn | 5 each | 64 | 0.7 | 0.4 | n/a | 13.7 | 5.0 |
| Cheddar Cheese | 6 each | 46 | 1.7 | 0.2 | n/a | 7.1 | 0.0 |
| Soy Crisps, White Cheddar, Trader Joe's | 18 | 110 | 3.0 | 0.0 | 0.0 | 14.0 | 1.0 |
| Sun Chips | 1 oz. | 140 | 6.0 | 0.5 | 0.0 | 19.0 | 2.0 |
| Taro Chips, Terra | 1 oz. | 140 | 6.0 | 0.5 | 0.0 | 19.0 | 2.0 |

## SOUPS

| Item | SERVING | CAL-ORIES | FAT GRAMS | SAT. FAT GRAMS | TRANS FAT GRAMS | CARB. GRAMS | SUGAR GRAMS |
|---|---|---|---|---|---|---|---|
| Asparagus, cream of | | | | | | | |
| Canned, prepared w/milk | 1 cup | 161 | 8.2 | 3.3 | 0.0 | 16.4 | n/a |
| Canned, prepared w/water | ½ cup | 110 | 7.0 | 2.0 | 0.0 | 9.0 | 2.0 |
| Bean and Bacon | 1 cup | 172 | 6.0 | 1.5 | 0.0 | 22.8 | 2.8 |
| Campbell's | ½ cup | 170 | 4.0 | 1.5 | 0.0 | 25.0 | 4.0 |
| ■ Healthy Choice | 1 cup | 150 | 2.0 | 0.5 | 0.0 | 28.0 | 4.0 |
| Beef & Barley | ½ cup | 90 | 1.5 | 1.0 | 0.0 | 15.0 | 2.0 |
| ■ Health Valley | 1 cup | 110 | 1.0 | 0.0 | 0.0 | 17.0 | 4.0 |
| Progresso | 1 cup | 140 | 1.0 | 0.0 | 0.0 | 22.0 | 4.0 |
| ■ 99% fat free | 1 each | 137 | 1.6 | 0.7 | n/a | 17.1 | n/a |
| Beef bouillon cube | ½ cube | 20 | 1.0 | 0.5 | 0.0 | <1 | 0.0 |
| Broth | 1 cup | 19 | 0.7 | 0.3 | 0.0 | 1.9 | 0.2 |
| ■ Beef consommé, prepared w/water | 1 cup | 29 | 0.0 | 0.0 | 0.0 | 1.8 | n/a |
| Beef Noodle, Progresso | 1 cup | 140 | 3.5 | 1.5 | n/a | 15.0 | 2.0 |
| ■ Black Bean Vegetable, Health Valley | 1 cup | 120 | 0.0 | 0.0 | 0.0 | 24.0 | 8.0 |
| Bouillon/Broth, chicken, 99% fat free, Swanson | 1 cup | 5 | 0.2 | 0.0 | 0.0 | 0.2 | 0.2 |
| Celery, cream of, condensed | ½ cup | 90 | 6.0 | 1.0 | 0.0 | 9.0 | 1.0 |
| ■ Chicken broth, homemade, low fat | 1 cup | 34 | 0.0 | 0.0 | 0.0 | n/a | n/a |
| ■ Campbell's low sodium | 1 cup | 25 | 0.5 | 0.5 | 0.0 | 1.0 | 1.0 |
| ■ Health Valley | 1 cup | 30 | 0.0 | 0.0 | 0.0 | 2.0 | 1.0 |
| Health Valley, no salt added | 1 cup | 35 | 1.5 | 0.5 | 0.0 | 0.0 | 0.0 |
| ■ Pritikin | 1 cup | 10 | 0.0 | 0.0 | 0.0 | <1 | 0.0 |
| Swanson | 1 cup | 15 | 0.5 | 0.0 | 0.0 | 1.0 | 1.0 |

■ Contains less than 20% fat
n/a Not available

* See note, page xli

| Item | SERVING | CAL-ORIES | FAT GRAMS | SAT. FAT GRAMS | TRANS FAT GRAMS | CARB. GRAMS | SUGAR GRAMS |
|---|---|---|---|---|---|---|---|
| Chicken, cream of, Campbell's | ½ cup | 120 | 8.0 | 0.0 | 0.0 | 10.0 | 1.0 |
| Healthy Request, condensed | ½ cup | 70 | 2.5 | 1.0 | 0.0 | 12.0 | 2.0 |
| Low sodium, Campbell's Cream of Chicken | ½ cup | 80 | 2.5 | 1.0 | 0.0 | 12.0 | 2.0 |
| ■ Chicken Gumbo, Campbell's | 1 cup | 60 | 1.0 | 0.5 | n/a | 10.0 | 2.0 |
| Chicken noodle | | | | | | | |
| Chunky, Campbell's | 1 cup | 120 | 2.5 | 1.0 | 0.0 | 15.0 | 2.0 |
| ■ Health Valley, in a cup | 1 serv. | 220 | 0.0 | 0.0 | 0.0 | 48.0 | 2.0 |
| ■ Healthy Choice | 1 cup | 100 | 1.5 | 0.0 | 0.0 | 13.0 | 1.0 |
| ■ Lipton Cup-a-Soup | 1 env. | 45 | 7.3 | 1.0 | 0.0 | 8.0 | 0.0 |
| ■ Nile Spice, in a cup | 1 serv. | 90 | 1.0 | 0.0 | n/a | 16.0 | 3.0 |
| ■ Progresso | 1 cup | 100 | 2.0 | 0.5 | 0.0 | 13.0 | 1.0 |
| W/dumplings, Tabatchnick | 1 cup | 70 | 2.0 | 0.0 | 0.0 | 27.0 | 5.0 |
| ■ Chicken, Grilled, Chunky | ½ cup | 100 | 2.0 | 0.5 | 0.0 | 15.0 | 2.0 |
| ■ Chicken Rice, Campbell's, condensed | ½ cup | 70 | 1.5 | 0.5 | 0.0 | 13.0 | 1.0 |
| ■ Health Valley | 1 cup | 130 | 2.0 | 0.0 | n/a | 21.0 | 4.0 |
| ■ Healthy Choice | 1 cup | 90 | 1.5 | 0.0 | 0.0 | 14 | 1.0 |
| Healthy Request | 1 cup | 62 | 2.0 | 0.6 | n/a | 8.6 | 0.5 |
| Manischewitz | 1 cup | 45 | 3.0 | 1.0 | n/a | 4.0 | 0.0 |
| Wild Rice, Progresso | 1 cup | 93 | 2.2 | 0.6 | 0.0 | 12.0 | n/a |
| ■ Chicken Vegetable, Progresso | 1 cup | 90 | 1.5 | 0.0 | 0.0 | 11.0 | 1.0 |
| Clam chowder, Manhattan, Progresso | 1 cup | 134 | 3.4 | 2.1 | n/a | 18.8 | 4.0 |
| Clam chowder, New England, Progresso | 1 cup | 190 | 10.0 | 2.5 | 0.0 | 20.0 | 3.0 |
| ■ 98% fat free, Campbell's | 1 cup | 110 | 1.5 | 0.5 | n/a | 19.0 | 2.0 |
| ■ Healthy Choice | 1 cup | 120 | 1.5 | 1.0 | 0.0 | 24.0 | 2.0 |
| Corn chowder, Campbell's | 1 cup | 230 | 13.0 | 3.0 | 0.0 | 19.0 | 3.0 |
| ■ w/chicken, Healthy Choice | 1 cup | 150 | 2.5 | 1.0 | 0.0 | 28.0 | 3.0 |
| ■ w/tomato, Health Valley | 1 cup | 200 | 0.0 | 0.0 | 0.0 | 42.0 | 2.0 |
| * ■ Fish Soup Mediterranean | 1.5 cups | 163 | 3.5 | 0.6 | 0.0 | n/a | n/a |
| ■ Four Bean, Manischewitz | 1 cup | 105 | 1.5 | 0.0 | 0.0 | 48.0 | n/a |
| * ■ Gazpacho | ¾ cup | 35 | 0.2 | 0.0 | 0.0 | n/a | n/a |
| Leek | 1 cup | 71 | 2.1 | 1.0 | n/a | 11.4 | 0.8 |
| * ■ Lentil, homemade | 1 cup | 158 | 0.4 | n/a | 0.0 | n/a | n/a |
| ■ Health Valley | 1 cup | 110 | 2.0 | 0.0 | 0.0 | 21.0 | 4.0 |
| ■ Progresso | 1 cup | 126 | 1.5 | 0.3 | 0.0 | 20.3 | n/a |
| ■ w/ham | 1 cup | 139 | 2.8 | 1.1 | 0.0 | 20.2 | n/a |
| ■ Lentil Curry Cous Cous, Nile Spice | 1 serv. | 200 | 1.5 | 0.0 | 0.0 | 36.0 | 5.0 |
| ■ Lentil Mediterranean, Westbrae Natural | 1 cup | 140 | 0.0 | 0.0 | 0.0 | 24.0 | 5.0 |
| Matzo Ball, Manischewitz | 1 cup | 110 | 5.0 | 2.0 | 0.0 | 13.0 | 1.0 |
| * Minestrone | | | | | | | |
| ■ Campbell's | 1 cup | 100 | 0.0 | 0.0 | 0.0 | 20.0 | 3.0 |
| ■ Health Valley | 1 cup | 110 | 0.0 | 0.0 | 0.0 | 23.0 | 6.0 |

■ Contains less than 20% fat
n/a Not available

* See note, page xli

| Item | SERVING | CAL-ORIES | FAT GRAMS | SAT. FAT GRAMS | TRANS FAT GRAMS | CARB. GRAMS | SUGAR GRAMS |
|---|---|---|---|---|---|---|---|
| ■ Healthy Choice | 1 cup | 120 | 1.5 | 0.0 | 0.0 | 26.0 | 7.0 |
| ■ Healthy Request, Campbell's | 1/2 cup | 80 | 0.5 | 0.0 | 0.0 | 15.0 | 4.0 |
| ■ Pritikin | 1 cup | 90 | 0.0 | 0.0 | 0.0 | 18.0 | 3.0 |
| ■ Progresso | 1 cup | 120 | 1.5 | 0.0 | 0.0 | 22.0 | 4.0 |
| ■ Tabatchnick | 1 cup | 120 | 1.0 | 0.0 | 0.0 | 24.0 | 3.0 |
| ■ Minestrone Cous Cous, Nile Spice | 1 serv. | 180 | 1.5 | 0.0 | 0.0 | 34.0 | 7.0 |
| Mushroom, cream of | | | | | | | |
| Campbell's | 1/2 cup | 100 | 6.0 | 1.5 | 0.0 | 9.0 | 1.0 |
| Low sodium, low fat, Healthy Request | 1/2 cup | 70 | 2.5 | 1.0 | 0.0 | 10.0 | 2.0 |
| Lipton Cup-a-Soup | 1 serv. | 4 | 0.1 | 0.0 | 0.0 | 0.7 | 0.1 |
| Progresso | 1 cup | 90 | 2.0 | 0.5 | 0.0 | 12.0 | 2.0 |
| Westbrae Natural | 1 cup | 93 | 4.0 | 2.0 | 0.0 | 13.3 | 0.0 |
| Mushroom Barley, Health Valley | 1 cup | 90 | 2.0 | 0.0 | 0.0 | 17.0 | 4.0 |
| Streit's | 1 cup | 80 | 1.5 | 0.0 | 0.0 | 14.0 | 3.0 |
| Onion | 1 cup | 113 | 3.5 | 0.5 | 0.0 | 16.4 | 2.6 |
| French, Campbell's | 1 cup | 45 | 1.5 | 0.5 | 0.0 | 6.0 | <1 |
| Oriental Ramen Noodle | 1/2 pkg. | 190 | 7.0 | 3.5 | 0.0 | 26 | <1 |
| Oxtail | 1 cup | 71 | 2.6 | 1.3 | n/a | 9.0 | 2.7 |
| Oyster stew | 1 cup | 80 | 6.0 | 3.5 | n/a | 5.0 | 0.0 |
| Potato, cream of | 1/2 cup | 90 | 2.0 | 1.0 | 0.0 | 15.0 | 1.0 |
| Shrimp, cream of | 1 cup | 90 | 6.0 | 2.0 | n/a | 8.0 | 1.0 |
| Shrimp, Ramen | 1/2 pkg. | 190 | 7.0 | 3.5 | 0.0 | 26 | <1 |
| ■ Split Pea | 1 cup | 180 | 2.3 | 0.8 | 0.0 | 29.9 | 8.8 |
| ■ Amy's | 1 cup | 100 | 0.0 | 0.0 | 0.0 | 19.0 | 4.0 |
| ■ w/ham, Healthy Choice | 1 cup | 170 | 2.0 | 0.5 | 0.0 | 25 | 4.0 |
| w/ham, Progresso | 1 cup | 150 | 1.0 | 0.5 | 0.0 | 25 | 4.0 |
| ■ Pritikin | 1 cup | 180 | 0.5 | 0.0 | 0.0 | 32.0 | 3.0 |
| ■ Tomato | 1 cup | 100 | 0.5 | 0.5 | 0.0 | 21.0 | 12.0 |
| ■ w/basil, Progresso | 1 cup | 160 | 3.0 | 0.5 | 0.0 | 30 | 16.0 |
| ■ Chunky, Healthy Valley | 1 cup | 80 | 0.0 | 0.0 | 0.0 | 18.0 | 11.0 |
| ■ Garden, Campbell's Select | 1 cup | 100 | 0.5 | 0.5 | 0.0 | 21 | 12.0 |
| Tomato, beef & noodle | 1 cup | 139 | 4.3 | 1.6 | 0.0 | 21.2 | 2.6 |
| Tomato Bisque, Campbell's | 1/2 cup | 130 | 3.5 | 1.5 | 0.0 | 23.0 | 15.0 |
| ■ Tomato Rice, Campbell's | 1 cup | 110 | 2.0 | 0.5 | 0.0 | 23.0 | 10.0 |
| ■ Tomato & Rotini, Progresso | 1 cup | 130 | 1.6 | 0.0 | 0.0 | 23.8 | 6.5 |
| Tomato Vegetable, Progress | 1 cup | 90 | 2.0 | 0.0 | 0.0 | 15.0 | 8.0 |
| ■ Health Valley | 1 cup | 80 | 0.0 | 0.0 | 0.0 | 17.0 | 9.0 |
| ■ Turkey Noodle, Progresso | 1 cup | 100 | 0.5 | 0.0 | 0.0 | 14 | 1.0 |
| ■ Turkey Rice, Progresso | 1 cup | 110 | 1.0 | 0.0 | 0.0 | 18.0 | 2.0 |
| ■ Healthy Choice | 1 cup | 102 | 1.5 | 0.0 | 0.0 | 17.4 | 4.1 |
| * Vegetable | | | | | | | |
| Campbell's | 1 cup | 90 | 0.5 | 0.0 | 0.0 | 18.0 | 6.0 |
| Country, Healthy Choice | 1 cup | 100 | 0.0 | 0.0 | 0.0 | 22.0 | 5.0 |
| Country Vegetable, Healthy Choice | 1 cup | 110 | 1.0 | 0.0 | 0.0 | 19.0 | 4.0 |

■ Contains less than 20% fat
n/a Not available

* See note, page xli

| Item | SERVING | CAL-ORIES | FAT GRAMS | SAT. FAT GRAMS | TRANS FAT GRAMS | CARB. GRAMS | SUGAR GRAMS |
|---|---|---|---|---|---|---|---|
| Vegetarian Vegetable Alphabet, Campbell's | ½ cup | 90 | 5.0 | 0.0 | 0.0 | 18.0 | 6.0 |
| ■ Manischewitz | 1 cup | 140 | 3.0 | 0.0 | 0.0 | 26.0 | 8.0 |
| ■ Vegetarian, Pritikin | 1 cup | 80 | 0.0 | 0.0 | 0.0 | 15.0 | 0.0 |
| ■ Vegetable Barley, low fat, Amy's | 1 cup | 50 | 1.0 | 0.0 | 0.0 | 10.0 | 4.0 |
| ■ in a cup, Progresso | 1 cup | 80 | 0.5 | 0.0 | 0.0 | 17.0 | 3.0 |
| ■ Vegetable Beef, Progresso | 1 cup | 120 | 1.0 | 0.0 | 0.0 | 20.0 | 5.0 |
| Chunky, Campbell's | 1 cup | 130 | 2.5 | 1.0 | 0.0 | 18.0 | 4.0 |
| ■ Vegetable broth, Imagine | 1 cup | 30 | 0.0 | 0.0 | 0.0 | 5.0 | 3.0 |
| ■ Swanson | 1 cup | 15 | 0.0 | 0.0 | 0.0 | 3.0 | 2.0 |
| Wonton | 1 serv. | 52 | 3.0 | 1.0 | 0.0 | 4.0 | n/a |

## SPICES & CONDIMENTS

| Item | SERVING | CAL-ORIES | FAT GRAMS | SAT. FAT GRAMS | TRANS FAT GRAMS | CARB. GRAMS | SUGAR GRAMS |
|---|---|---|---|---|---|---|---|
| ■ Curry paste, red | 1 tb. | 10 | 0.0 | 0.0 | 0.0 | n/a | n/a |
| Curry powder | 1 tsp. | 7 | 0.3 | 0.0 | 0.0 | 1.2 | 0.1 |
| ■ Garlic powder | 1 tsp. | 9 | 0.0 | 0.0 | 0.0 | 2.0 | 0.7 |
| ■ Horseradish, prepared | 1 tsp. | 2 | 0.0 | 0.0 | 0.0 | 0.6 | 0.4 |
| Ketchup | | | | | | | |
| ■ Annie's Natural | 1 tb. | 15 | 0.0 | 0.0 | 0.0 | 3.0 | 2.0 |
| ■ Heinz | 1 tb. | 15 | 0.0 | 0.0 | 0.0 | 4.0 | 4.0 |
| ■ Muir Glen | 1 tb. | 20 | 0.0 | 0.0 | 0.0 | 4.0 | 3.0 |
| Mayonnaise (see Salad Dressings) | | | | | | | |
| Miso, fermented soybean | 1 tb. | 34 | 1.0 | 0.2 | 0.0 | 4.6 | 1.1 |
| Mustard | | | | | | | |
| Grey Poupon, dijon | 1 tsp. | 6 | 0.5 | 0.0 | 0.0 | 0.6 | n/a |
| ■ Gulden's spicy brown | 1 tsp. | 0 | 0.0 | 0.0 | 0.0 | 0.0 | 0.0 |
| ■ Westbrae Natural, dijon | 1 tsp. | 0 | 0.0 | 0.0 | 0.0 | 0.0 | 0.0 |
| Olives, black, large, no pits | 2 each | 10 | 0.9 | 0.1 | 0.0 | 0.6 | 0.0 |
| Green, stuffed | 2 each | 8 | 0.9 | 0.1 | 0.0 | 0.2 | 0.0 |
| Calamata, no pits | 2 each | 21 | 2.0 | 0.2 | 0.0 | 0.7 | 0.0 |
| ■ Pickles, bread & butter, Vlasic | 1 oz. | 30 | 0.0 | 0.0 | 0.0 | 7.1 | 7.1 |
| ■ Dill | 1 each | 23 | 0.0 | 0.0 | 0.0 | 4.0 | 2.0 |
| ■ Sweet | 1 each | 29 | 0.1 | 0.0 | 0.0 | 8.0 | 0.9 |
| ■ Pickle relish, sweet | 1 tb. | 20 | 0.1 | 0.0 | 0.0 | 5.4 | 0.5 |
| Sour | 1 tb. | 3 | 0.1 | n/a | 0.0 | n/a | n/a |
| ■ Pimientos, canned | 2 tb. | 6 | 0.1 | 0.0 | 0.0 | 1.2 | 0.7 |
| Shake 'N Bake, original, for chicken | ⅛ packet | 40 | 1.0 | 0.0 | 0.0 | 7.0 | 1.0 |
| Tangy honey | ⅛ each | 45 | 1.0 | 0.0 | 0.0 | 9.0 | 6.0 |
| ■ Vinegar, balsamic | 1 tb. | 10 | 0.0 | n/a | 0.0 | 2.3 | 2.2 |
| ■ Apple cider | 1 tb. | 1 | 0.0 | n/a | 0.0 | 0.1 | 0.0 |
| Rice, natural, Nakano | 1 tb. | 0 | 0.0 | 0.0 | 0.0 | 0.0 | 0.0 |
| ■ Rice, seasoned, Nakano | 1 tb. | 12 | 0.0 | 0.0 | 0.0 | 3.0 | 3.0 |
| ■ Rice, wine, oriental, Vintage Lites | 1 tb. | 15 | 0.0 | 0.0 | 0.0 | 4.0 | 3.5 |
| Raspberry blush, Vintage Lites | 1 tb. | 20 | 0.0 | 0.0 | 0.0 | 5.0 | 5.0 |
| ■ Vinegar, white wine | 1 tb. | 5 | 0.0 | 0.0 | 0.0 | 1.0 | 0.0 |

■ Contains less than 20% fat
n/a Not available

| Item | SERVING | CAL-ORIES | FAT GRAMS | SAT. FAT GRAMS | TRANS FAT GRAMS | CARB. GRAMS | SUGAR GRAMS |
|---|---|---|---|---|---|---|---|

## VEGETABLES & BEANS

**Beans & Bean Products**

| Item | SERVING | CAL-ORIES | FAT GRAMS | SAT. FAT GRAMS | TRANS FAT GRAMS | CARB. GRAMS | SUGAR GRAMS |
|---|---|---|---|---|---|---|---|
| ■ Baked, vegetarian, canned | 1/2 cup | 119 | 0.5 | 0.1 | 0.0 | 26.9 | 11.5 |
| ■ w/pork | 1/2 cup | 134 | 2.0 | 0.8 | 0.0 | 25.3 | n/a |
| ■ Barbecue, B&M | 1/2 cup | 170 | 1.0 | 0.0 | 0.0 | 33.0 | 12.0 |
| ■ Black | 1/2 cup | 114 | 0.5 | 0.1 | 0.0 | 20.4 | n/a |
| ■ Broad | 1/2 cup | 94 | 0.3 | 0.1 | 0.0 | 16.7 | 1.6 |
| ■ Cannellini | 1/2 cup | 100 | 0.5 | 0.0 | 0.0 | 18.0 | 0.0 |
| ■ Chickpeas/garbanzos | 1/2 cup | 134 | 2.1 | 0.2 | 0.0 | 22.5 | 3.9 |
| ■ Cowpeas | 1/2 cup | 99 | 0.5 | 0.1 | 0.0 | 17.8 | 2.8 |
| ■ Great northern | 1/2 cup | 104 | 0.4 | 0.1 | 0.0 | 18.7 | n/a |
| Hummus | 1/2 cup | 208 | 12.0 | 1.8 | 0.0 | 17.9 | n/a |
| ■ Kidney | 1/2 cup | 112 | 0.4 | 0.1 | 0.0 | 20.2 | 0.3 |
| ■ Lentils | 1/2 cup | 115 | 0.4 | 0.1 | 0.0 | 19.9 | 1.8 |
| ■ Lima, baby, frozen | 1/2 cup | 95 | 0.3 | 0.1 | 0.0 | 17.5 | 1.2 |
| Fordhook, frozen | 1/2 cup | 99 | 0.3 | 0.1 | 0.0 | 18.6 | 2.6 |
| ■ Mature | 1/2 cup | 108 | 0.4 | 0.1 | 0.0 | 19.6 | 2.7 |
| ■ Mung | 1/2 cup | 106 | 0.4 | 0.1 | 0.0 | 19.3 | 2.0 |
| ■ Pinto | 1/2 cup | 122 | 0.6 | 0.1 | 0.0 | 22.4 | 0.3 |
| ■ Red | 1/2 cup | 100 | 0.0 | 0.0 | 0.0 | 19.0 | 2.0 |
| ■ Refried | 1/2 cup | 150 | 3.0 | 1.0 | 0.0 | 24.0 | 0.0 |
| Fat free | 1/2 cup | 110 | 0.0 | 0.0 | 0.0 | 21.0 | 1.0 |
| Soybeans, edamame | 1/2 cup | 100 | 2.5 | 0.0 | 0.0 | 9.0 | 2.0 |
| Soybeans, mature | 1/2 cup | 149 | 7.7 | 1.1 | 0.0 | 8.5 | 2.6 |
| ■ Split peas | 1/2 cup | 116 | 0.4 | 0.1 | 0.0 | 20.7 | 2.8 |
| Tempeh | 3 oz. | 168 | 9.7 | 2.9 | 0.0 | 8.0 | n/a |
| Tofu, raw, firm | 3 oz. | 84 | 5.6 | 0.9 | 0.0 | 0.9 | 0.0 |
| Silken | 3 oz. | 53 | 2.3 | 0.4 | 0.0 | 2.0 | 1.1 |
| ■ Light | 3 oz. | 31 | 0.7 | 0.1 | 0.0 | 0.9 | 0.4 |
| Soft | 3 oz. | 47 | 2.3 | 0.3 | 0.0 | 2.5 | 1.1 |
| ■ White | 1/2 cup | 124 | 0.3 | 0.1 | 0.0 | 22.5 | 0.3 |

**Vegetables & Potatoes**

| Item | SERVING | CAL-ORIES | FAT GRAMS | SAT. FAT GRAMS | TRANS FAT GRAMS | CARB. GRAMS | SUGAR GRAMS |
|---|---|---|---|---|---|---|---|
| Alfalfa sprouts | 1/2 cup | 5 | 0.1 | 0.0 | 0.0 | 0.6 | 0.0 |
| ■ Artichokes, fresh | 1 | 60 | 0.2 | 0.0 | 0.0 | 13.4 | 1.2 |
| ■ Frozen | 1/2 cup | 38 | 0.4 | 0.1 | 0.0 | 7.7 | 0.7 |
| ■ Artichoke hearts, canned | 1/2 cup | 38 | 0.0 | 0.0 | 0.0 | 6.3 | 0.0 |
| Arugula, fresh | 1/2 cup | 3 | 0.1 | 0.0 | 0.0 | 0.4 | 0.2 |
| ■ Asparagus, fresh, spears, cooked | 1 | 3 | 0.0 | 0.0 | 0.0 | 0.6 | 0.2 |
| Canned | 1/2 cup | 23 | 0.8 | 0.2 | 0.0 | 3.0 | 1.2 |
| ■ Bamboo shoots, fresh | 1/2 cup | 20 | 0.2 | 0.1 | 0.0 | 3.9 | 2.3 |
| ■ Beans, green, snap, cooked | 1/2 cup | 22 | 0.2 | 0.0 | 0.0 | 4.9 | 1.0 |
| ■ Canned | 1/2 cup | 14 | 0.1 | 0.0 | 0.0 | 3.0 | 0.7 |
| ■ Frozen | 1/2 cup | 19 | 0.1 | 0.0 | 0.0 | 4.4 | 0.8 |
| ■ Beans, yellow, snap, cooked | 1/2 cup | 22 | 0.2 | 0.0 | 0.0 | 4.9 | 1.0 |

■ Contains less than 20% fat
n/a Not available

| Item | SERVING | CAL-ORIES | FAT GRAMS | SAT. FAT GRAMS | TRANS FAT GRAMS | CARB. GRAMS | SUGAR GRAMS |
|---|---|---|---|---|---|---|---|
| ▪ Canned | ½ cup | 14 | 0.1 | 0.0 | 0.0 | 3.0 | 0.7 |
| ▪ Frozen | ½ cup | 19 | 0.1 | 0.0 | 0.0 | 4.4 | 0.8 |
| ▪ Beets, fresh, cooked | 1 | 22 | 0.1 | 0.0 | 0.0 | 5.0 | 4.0 |
| ▪ Canned | ½ cup | 26 | 0.1 | 0.0 | 0.0 | 6.1 | 4.7 |
| ▪ Pickled | ½ cup | 65 | 0.0 | 0.0 | 0.0 | 17.4 | 13.0 |
| ▪ Bok choy | ½ cup | 11 | 0.2 | 0.0 | 0.0 | 1.9 | 0.4 |
| ▪ Broccoli, florets, fresh, raw | ½ cup | 10 | 0.1 | 0.0 | 0.0 | 1.9 | n/a |
| ▪ Fresh, cooked | ½ cup | 22 | 0.3 | 0.0 | 0.0 | 4.0 | 1.1 |
| ▪ Frozen | ½ cup | 20 | 0.2 | 0.0 | 0.0 | 3.7 | 1.0 |
| ▪ Brussels sprouts, fresh, cooked | ½ cup | 28 | 0.4 | 0.1 | 0.0 | 5.5 | 1.4 |
| Cabbage | | | | | | | |
| ▪ Chinese, cooked | ½ cup | 10 | 0.1 | 0.0 | 0.0 | 1.5 | 0.7 |
| ▪ Green, cooked | ½ cup | 17 | 0.3 | 0.0 | 0.0 | 3.3 | 2.0 |
| ▪ Green, raw | ½ cup | 8 | 0.0 | 0.0 | 0.0 | 2.0 | 1.2 |
| ▪ Red, cooked | ½ cup | 22 | 0.1 | 0.0 | 0.0 | 5.2 | 2.5 |
| ▪ Red, raw | ½ cup | 11 | 0.1 | 0.0 | 0.0 | 2.6 | 1.4 |
| ▪ Carrots, cooked | ½ cup | 27 | 0.1 | 0.0 | 0.0 | 6.4 | 2.7 |
| ▪ Raw | 1 | 25 | 0.2 | 0.0 | 0.0 | 5.8 | 2.8 |
| ▪ Cauliflower, cooked | ½ cup | 14 | 0.3 | 0.0 | 0.0 | 2.6 | 0.9 |
| ▪ Raw | ½ cup | 13 | 0.1 | 0.0 | 0.0 | 2.7 | 1.2 |
| ▪ Frozen | ½ cup | 17 | 0.2 | 0.0 | 0.0 | 3.4 | 0.9 |
| ▪ Celeriac, cooked | ½ cup | 21 | 0.2 | 0.0 | 0.0 | 4.6 | n/a |
| ▪ Celery, cooked | ½ cup | 14 | 0.1 | 0.0 | 0.0 | 3.0 | 1.8 |
| ▪ Raw, chopped | ½ cup | 8 | 0.1 | 0.0 | 0.0 | 1.8 | 0.9 |
| ▪ Raw, stalk | 1 | 10 | 0.0 | 0.0 | 0.0 | 2.5 | 0.0 |
| ▪ Chayote, cooked | ½ cup | 19 | 0.4 | 0.1 | 0.0 | 4.1 | n/a |
| Collard greens (see Greens) | | | | | | | |
| Corn | | | | | | | |
| ▪ Baby | 5 | 43 | 0.5 | 0.1 | 0.0 | 10.0 | 1.3 |
| ▪ Canned | ½ cup | 106 | 0.0 | 0.0 | 0.0 | 22.7 | 6.1 |
| ▪ Cream style | ½ cup | 100 | 0.5 | 0.0 | 0.0 | 22.0 | 11.0 |
| ▪ On the cob | 1 | 83 | 1.0 | 0.2 | 0.0 | 19.3 | 2.4 |
| ▪ Shoepeg, canned | ½ cup | 121 | 0.8 | 0.0 | 0.0 | 24.2 | 4.6 |
| ▪ Sweet, cooked | ½ cup | 89 | 1.1 | 0.2 | 0.0 | 20.6 | 2.6 |
| ▪ Cucumber, fresh | 1 | 24 | 0.3 | 0.0 | 0.0 | 4.3 | 2.8 |
| ▪ Eggplant, cooked, cubed | ½ cup | 17 | 0.1 | 0.0 | 0.0 | 4.3 | 1.6 |
| ▪ Stir fried | ½ cup | 53 | 4.0 | 0.5 | 0.0 | 2.0 | 1.5 |
| ▪ Endive, Belgian, fresh | ½ cup | 8 | 0.0 | 0.0 | 0.0 | 1.8 | n/a |
| ▪ Escarole, fresh | ½ cup | 4 | 0.1 | 0.0 | 0.0 | 0.8 | 0.1 |
| ▪ Fennel, fresh | ½ cup | 13 | 0.1 | 0.0 | 0.0 | 3.2 | 0.1 |
| ▪ Garlic, fresh | 1 tsp. | 4 | 0.0 | 0.0 | 0.0 | 1.0 | 0.1 |
| ▪ Ginger root, fresh | 1 tsp. | 2 | 0.0 | 0.0 | 0.0 | 0.4 | 0.0 |
| Greens | | | | | | | |
| ▪ Beet, cooked | ½ cup | 19 | 0.1 | 0.0 | 0.0 | 3.9 | 0.4 |
| ▪ Collard, cooked | ½ cup | 25 | 0.3 | 0.0 | 0.0 | 4.7 | 0.4 |
| ▪ Dandelion, cooked | ½ cup | 17 | 0.3 | 0.1 | 0.0 | 3.4 | 1.4 |
| ▪ Kale, cooked | ½ cup | 18 | 0.3 | 0.0 | 0.0 | 3.7 | 0.8 |

▪ Contains less than 20% fat
n/a Not available

| Item | SERVING | CAL-ORIES | FAT GRAMS | SAT. FAT GRAMS | TRANS FAT GRAMS | CARB. GRAMS | SUGAR GRAMS |
|---|---|---|---|---|---|---|---|
| ■ Mustard, cooked | 1/2 cup | 11 | 0.2 | 0.0 | 0.0 | 1.5 | 0.1 |
| ■ Swiss chard, cooked | 1/2 cup | 18 | 0.1 | 0.0 | 0.0 | 3.6 | 1.0 |
| ■ Turnip, cooked | 1/2 cup | 14 | 0.2 | 0.0 | 0.0 | 3.1 | 0.4 |
| ■ Hearts of palm, canned | 1/2 cup | 20 | 0.5 | 0.1 | 0.0 | 3.4 | n/a |
| ■ Jerusalem artichoke, fresh | 1/2 cup | 57 | 0.0 | 0.0 | 0.0 | 13.1 | 7.2 |
| ■ Jicama, cooked | 1/2 cup | 19 | 0.0 | 0.0 | 0.0 | 4.4 | n/a |
| ■ Kohlrabi, cooked | 1/2 cup | 24 | 0.1 | 0.0 | 0.0 | 5.5 | 2.3 |
| ■ Leeks, cooked | 1/2 cup | 16 | 0.1 | 0.0 | 0.0 | 4.0 | 0.5 |
| Lettuce | | | | | | | |
| ■ Butterhead | 1/2 cup | 4 | 0.1 | 0.0 | 0.0 | 0.6 | 0.3 |
| ■ Iceberg | 1/2 cup | 4 | 0.0 | 0.0 | 0.0 | 0.8 | 0.5 |
| ■ Looseleaf | 1/2 cup | 4 | 0.0 | 0.0 | 0.0 | 0.8 | 0.2 |
| ■ Romaine | 1/2 cup | 5 | 0.1 | 0.0 | 0.0 | 0.9 | 0.3 |
| ■ Lotus root, cooked | 1/2 cup | 40 | 0.0 | 0.0 | 0.0 | 9.6 | 0.3 |
| ■ Mixed vegetables, frozen, Bird's Eye | 1/2 cup | 79 | 0.5 | 0.1 | 0.0 | 17.5 | 4.8 |
| Oriental | 1/2 cup | 41 | 0.8 | 0.2 | 0.0 | 6.6 | 1.9 |
| ■ Mushrooms, button, fresh | 1/2 cup | 8 | 0.1 | 0.0 | 0.0 | 1.1 | 0.7 |
| ■ Canned | 1/2 cup | 20 | 0.2 | 0.0 | 0.0 | 4.0 | 1.7 |
| Portabella | 1 | 27 | 0.1 | n/a | 0.0 | 4.3 | 1.5 |
| ■ Okra, cooked | 1/2 cup | 18 | 0.1 | 0.0 | 0.0 | 3.6 | 1.8 |
| ■ Onions, raw, chopped | 1/2 cup | 34 | 0.1 | 0.0 | 0.0 | 8.1 | 3.4 |
| Onion rings | 1 serv. | 320 | 16.0 | 4.0 | n/a | 39.0 | 4.0 |
| Onion rings, canned, French's | 3 oz. | 530 | 40.7 | 10.2 | n/a | 33.9 | 0.5 |
| ■ Parsley, fresh | 1/2 cup | 11 | 0.2 | 0.0 | 0.0 | 1.9 | 0.3 |
| ■ Parsnips, cooked | 1/2 cup | 55 | 0.2 | 0.0 | 0.0 | 13.3 | 3.7 |
| ■ Peas, green, cooked | 1/2 cup | 67 | 0.2 | 0.0 | 0.0 | 12.5 | 4.7 |
| ■ Snow, cooked | 1/2 cup | 35 | 0.2 | 0.0 | 0.0 | 6.3 | 3.3 |
| ■ Sugar snap, cooked | 1/2 cup | 38 | 0.0 | 0.0 | 0.0 | 7.6 | 3.8 |
| ■ Peas & carrots, frozen, | 1/2 cup | 38 | 0.3 | 0.1 | 0.0 | 8.1 | 3.5 |
| ■ Peppers, bell, red or green, fresh | 1/2 cup | 15 | 0.1 | 0.0 | 0.0 | 3.5 | 1.8 |
| ■ Cooked | 1/2 cup | 19 | 0.1 | 0.0 | 0.0 | 4.6 | 2.3 |
| ■ Hot chili | 1/2 cup | 14 | 0.3 | 0.0 | 0.0 | 2.7 | 1.5 |
| ■ Pimiento, canned | 1/2 cup | 22 | 0.3 | 0.0 | 0.0 | 4.9 | 2.8 |
| ■ Poi | 1/2 cup | 134 | 0.2 | 0.0 | 0.0 | 32.7 | 0.5 |
| Potatoes | | | | | | | |
| Au gratin | 1 | 127 | 5.6 | 3.5 | n/a | 17.6 | n/a |
| ■ Baked, w/skin | 6 oz. | 128 | 0.2 | 0.1 | 0.0 | 29.1 | 1.6 |
| ■ Boiled, diced | 1/2 cup | 67 | 0.1 | 0.0 | 0.0 | 15.6 | 0.7 |
| Mashed w/milk & butter | 1/2 cup | 119 | 4.4 | 1.8 | 0.1 | 17.6 | 0.8 |
| *■ Roast potatoes w/basil | 1 serv. | 136 | 1.5 | 0.3 | 0.0 | n/a | n/a |
| Pancakes | 1 | 207 | 11.6 | 2.3 | 0.0 | 21.8 | n/a |
| Puffs | 1/2 cup | 113 | 5.5 | 2.6 | n/a | 15.6 | n/a |
| Scalloped | 1 serv. | 30 | 0.7 | n/a | n/a | 5.3 | n/a |
| ■ Scalloped, cheesy | 1/2 cup | 110 | 1.5 | 0.0 | n/a | 22.0 | 2.0 |
| Potatoes, frozen, Ore-Ida French fries, crinkle cut | 3 oz. | 190 | 3.6 | 1.0 | 1.5 | 20.2 | 0.5 |

■ Contains less than 20% fat
n/a Not available

* See note, page xli

| Item | SERVING | CAL-ORIES | FAT GRAMS | SAT. FAT GRAMS | TRANS FAT GRAMS | CARB. GRAMS | SUGAR GRAMS |
|---|---|---|---|---|---|---|---|
| Hash browns | 1/2 cup | 62 | 4.8 | 1.9 | 0.0 | 13.8 | n/a |
| Snackin' fries | 3 oz. | 204 | 12.0 | 2.1 | n/a | 21.6 | 1.8 |
| Tater tots | 9 pieces | 150 | 6.0 | 1.0 | 0.0 | 21.0 | 0.5 |
| ■ Potatoes, sweet, baked, w/skin | 6 oz. | 93 | 0.2 | 0.1 | 0.0 | 21.4 | 8.7 |
| ■ Candied | 1/2 cup | 276 | 0.8 | 0.4 | 0.0 | 66.9 | 45.1 |
| ■ Mashed | 1/2 cup | 125 | 0.2 | 0.1 | 0.0 | 29.1 | 9.4 |
| ■ Pumpkin, canned | 1/2 cup | 42 | 0.3 | 0.2 | 0.0 | 9.9 | 4.0 |
| ■ Radicchio, fresh | 1/2 cup | 5 | 0.1 | 0.0 | 0.0 | 0.9 | 0.1 |
| ■ Radishs, fresh | 1/2 cup | 9 | 0.1 | 0.0 | 0.0 | 2.0 | 1.1 |
| ■ Rutabaga, cooked | 1/2 cup | 33 | 0.2 | 0.0 | 0.0 | 7.4 | 5.1 |
| ■ Sauerkraut, canned | 1/2 cup | 16 | 0.0 | 0.0 | 0.0 | 4.0 | 0.0 |
| ■ Scallions, fresh | 1/2 cup | 16 | 0.1 | 0.0 | 0.0 | 3.7 | 1.2 |
| ■ Seaweed, kelp, fresh | 1/2 cup | 17 | 0.2 | 0.1 | 0.0 | 3.8 | 0.2 |
| ■ Shallots, fresh | 2 tb. | 14 | 0.0 | 0.0 | 0.0 | 3.4 | 0.6 |
| ■ Spinach, fresh | 1/2 cup | 3 | 0.1 | 0.0 | 0.0 | 0.5 | 0.1 |
| ■ Cooked | 1/2 cup | 21 | 0.2 | 0.0 | 0.0 | 3.4 | 0.4 |
| Creamed, Bird's Eye | 1/2 cup | 111 | 8.0 | 4.6 | 0.0 | 7.4 | 4.4 |
| Squash | | | | | | | |
| ■ Acorn, baked, cubed | 1/2 cup | 57 | 0.1 | 0.0 | 0.0 | 14.9 | n/a |
| ■ Mashed | 1/2 cup | 42 | 0.1 | 0.0 | 0.0 | 10.8 | n/a |
| ■ Butternut, baked, cubed | 1/2 cup | 41 | 0.1 | 0.0 | 0.0 | 10.8 | 2.0 |
| ■ Mashed | 1/2 cup | 47 | 0.1 | 0.0 | 0.0 | 12.1 | 4.9 |
| ■ Hubbard, baked, cubed | 1/2 cup | 60 | 0.7 | 0.2 | 0.0 | 13.0 | n/a |
| ■ Mashed | 1/2 cup | 35 | 0.4 | 0.1 | 0.0 | 7.6 | 3.5 |
| ■ Spaghetti, cooked | 1/2 cup | 21 | 0.2 | 0.1 | 0.0 | 5.0 | 2.0 |
| ■ Summer, cooked | 1/2 cup | 18 | 0.3 | 0.1 | 0.0 | 3.9 | 2.3 |
| ■ Zucchini, cooked | 1/2 cup | 13 | 0.1 | 0.0 | 0.0 | 2.6 | 1.5 |
| ■ Succotash, frozen | 1/2 cup | 79 | 0.8 | 0.1 | 0.0 | 17.0 | 1.9 |
| ■ Taro, cooked | 1/2 cup | 30 | 0.5 | 0.1 | 0.0 | 4.7 | n/a |
| Tomatillo, fresh | 1/2 cup | 21 | 0.7 | 0.1 | 0.0 | 3.9 | 2.6 |
| ■ Tomatoes, fresh | 1 | 35 | 0.5 | 0.0 | 0.0 | 7.0 | 4.0 |
| ■ Cherry | 1/2 cup | 13 | 0.2 | 0.0 | 0.0 | 2.9 | 2.0 |
| Canned | | | | | | | |
| ■ Diced, Muir Glen | 1/2 cup | 25 | 0.0 | 0.0 | 0.0 | 4.4 | 3.1 |
| ■ Diced, unsalted, Del Monte | 1/2 cup | 25 | 0.0 | 0.0 | 0.0 | 6.0 | 4.0 |
| ■ Crushed, San Marzanno | 1/4 cup | 25 | 0.0 | 0.0 | 0.0 | 7.0 | 3.0 |
| ■ Paste, Contadina | 2 tb. | 30 | 0.0 | 0.0 | 0.0 | 6.0 | 3.0 |
| ■ Pureed, Progresso | 1/2 cup | 50 | 0.0 | 0.0 | 0.0 | 10.0 | 6.0 |
| ■ Whole, peeled, Muir Glen | 1/2 cup | 28 | 0.0 | 0.0 | 0.0 | 4.8 | 3.5 |
| ■ Turnips, fresh | 1/2 cup | 18 | 0.1 | 0.0 | 0.0 | 4.2 | 2.5 |
| ■ Cooked | 1/2 cup | 17 | 0.1 | 0.0 | 0.0 | 4.0 | 2.3 |
| ■ Water chestnuts, sliced | 1/2 cup | 60 | 0.1 | 0.0 | 0.0 | 14.8 | 3.0 |
| ■ Watercress, fresh, chopped | 1/2 cup | 2 | 0.0 | 0.0 | 0.0 | 0.2 | 0.0 |
| ■ Yams, baked, cubed | 1/2 cup | 79 | 0.1 | 0.0 | 0.0 | 18.8 | 0.3 |

■ Contains less than 20% fat
n/a Not available